The Medical School Admissions Guide

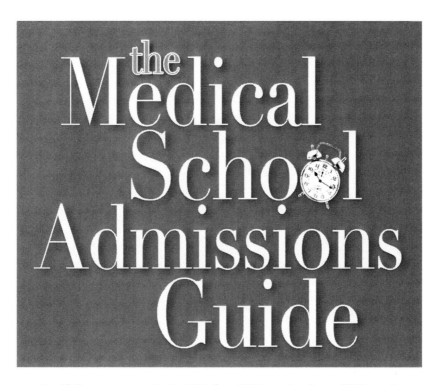

the Medical School Admissions Guide

A Harvard MD's Week-by-Week Admissions Handbook

3RD EDITION

Suzanne M. Miller, MD

Requests for permission to make copies of any part of the work should be e-mailed to:
info@MDadmit.com

www.MDadmit.com

The prices and rates stated in this book are subject to change.

Library of Congress Control Number 2014903384

ISBN 978-1-936633-80-7

Layout and cover design by Casey Hooper

Text set in Arno Pro

Printed in the United States of America

Also by Dr. Suzanne M. Miller

How to be Pre-Med: A Harvard MD's
Medical School Preparation Guide for Students and Parents

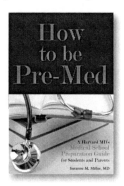

Available at amazon.com, barnesandnoble.com, and MDadmit.com

How To Get Into Medical School With A Low GPA

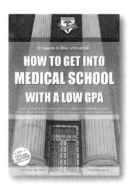

Available at howtobepremed.com

Acknowledgements

I would like to thank the MDadmit clients and friends who allowed their work to be reproduced for readers' benefit including Jason Aguirre, Phillip Carron, Lauren Katkish, Alyn Kelley, Madison Li, Akash Parekh, Michael Polignano, Megan Simon Thomas, Alexandra Weiss, Abigail Werner, Emmagene Worley, Rochelle Zarzar, Sara Wilson, and Stefani Su…Sharon Miller, gatekeeper of the terrible word "that," dangling modifiers, split infinitives, and other grammatical wonders, for her endless patience and hard work on the final draft… Jennifer Abbott for invaluable editing…Ron "Duck" Toole for vision behind the lens and skill behind the computer…Casey Hooper for a lovely cover and layout…Hannah Grausz and Jonathan Nielson for honest advice…Rich MacClary, Keith Zimmermann, Scott Talan, and Chris Kiple for counsel on all things business…Ria Reisner, Emma Philips, Nicki Gill, and Nils Olson for serving as sounding boards, sources of encouragement, and fabulous friends… Adam Elshaug , John Miller, Kristin MacClary, and Andrea Zimmermann for letting me talk for hours about the book to flesh out ideas…and all of those who dream of becoming doctors who make this book possible.

Table of Contents

Appendices

Preface

This guide contains the weekly, step-by-step plan I used to get into Harvard Medical School and have since utilized to help hundreds of applicants gain entry into medical school. Following this strategy will give you a distinct advantage in the medical school admissions process. Over 40,000 individuals apply to United States medical schools every year with less than half gaining admissions. It takes more than academic and extracurricular prowess to get into medical school.

Did you know:

- Recommendations should not all come from college science professors?
- The new MCAT arrives in 2015 and involves a whole new section?
- Transcripts should be ordered from your college or university months before the AMCAS application opens?
- Texas medical schools require a separate application called TMDSAS? And DO schools have their own application called AACOMAS?
- The AMCAS work/activities section is more than a resume?
- You may be required to write over 50 essays during the admissions cycle (AMCAS personal statement plus secondary essays)?

- Ethical and political questions are now standard in medical school interviews?
- The Multiple Mini Interview (MMI) is growing in popularity and requires different preparation than a traditional interview?

This week-by-week guide lays out all the insider tips I have learned over the past decade as a Harvard pre-med tutor, admissions interviewer, and medical school admissions consultant. I noticed one of the most difficult aspects of the medical school admissions process is knowing when to do what, so I created a handbook that breaks down the many tasks of medical school admissions into weekly themes and offers successful examples of medical school personal statements, work/activities, secondary essays, and letters of intent.. If you follow this guide, you will be prepared for every step in the process, hit each deadline with ease, and create your best application.

I also created this guide to offer my MDadmit clients an easily affordable admissions consulting option. I do know, however, that everyone's situation is different and that the most effective advice is personal. If you would like to use MDadmit's personal admissions consulting services, feel free to contact me at info@MDadmit.com.

Good luck and get in!

Dr. Miller

How to Use This Handbook

This guide is for individuals who have decided to apply to medical school. It will not help you determine whether medicine is the right career for you or evaluate whether you have the credentials to get into medical school. For such questions, speak with your pre-med advisor and/or an admissions consultant.

To gain the most from this guide, initially read it cover-to-cover so you understand the complexity of the medical school admissions process and know what to expect. Then, as you move through the admissions cycle, follow the week-by-week advice.

I certainly cannot guarantee you admission to medical school by reading this book and following its advice. But I can assure your chances of medical school admission success will improve by learning the details of the complex admissions process and using the insider tips.

Legal Disclaimer

The author/publisher of this book has used her best efforts in preparing this book. The author/publisher makes no representation or warranties with respect to the accuracy, applicability, fitness, or completeness of the contents of this book. The information contained in this book is strictly for educational purposes. Therefore, if you wish to apply ideas contained in this book, you are taking full responsibility for your actions. The author/publisher shall in no event be held liable to any party for any direct, indirect, punitive, special, incidental, or other consequential damages arising directly or indirectly from any use of this material, which is provided "as is" and without warranties.

The author/publisher does not warrant the performance, effectiveness, or applicability of any websites listed in this book. All websites are listed for information purposes only and are not warranted for content, accuracy, or any other implied or explicit purpose.

The author/publisher of this book made every effort to be as accurate and complete as possible in the creation of the book's content. However, due to the rapidly changing nature of medical school admissions, she does not warrant or represent at any time that the contents within are accurate. Application fees, dates, deadlines, and addresses, in addition to admissions requirements, change every year, and it is the reader's responsibility to stay up-to-date on such changes.

The author/publisher will not be responsible for any losses or damages of any kind incurred by the reader whether directly or indirectly arising from the use of the information found in this book.

Acronyms

The medical school admissions process and this book are full of acronyms. I've put them all in one place for easy reference.

AMCAS—American Medical College Application Service

TMDSAS—Texas Medical & Dental Schools Application Service

OMSAS—Ontario Medical Schools Application Service

AACOMAS—American Association of Colleges of Osteopathic Medicine Application Service

AAMC—Association of American Medical Colleges

AACOM—American Association of Colleges of Osteopathic Medicine

MCAT—Medical College Admission Test

FAP—Fee Assistance Program

MD—Doctor of Medicine

DO—Doctor of Osteopathy

MBA—Master of Business Administration

JD—Juris Doctor (Law)

MPH—Master of Public Health

MPA—Master of Public Administration

PhD—Doctor of Philosophy

USMLE—United States Medical Licensing Examination

January Year 1
Money and the MCAT

"The secret of getting ahead is getting started. The secret of getting started is breaking your complex overwhelming tasks into small manageable tasks, and then starting on the first one."
-MARK TWAIN

Happy New Year! What better way to kick off a new year than to begin the medical school application cycle? Sure, you could spend the winter vacation skiing in Tahoe, relaxing in the Bahamas, or trekking in the Outback. But you've decided to become a doctor and it's time to get going. "But medical school is more than a year away," you say. In fact, it's 21 months away. Seems far off, but preparing a successful application without becoming a total stress case takes a good long time. The medical application process is difficult because there are so many hoops to jump through. But as long as you are well versed on the expectations and deadlines of medical school admissions, you will survive this hectic process with time left over to enjoy that dream vacation and hopefully get one-step closer to doctorhood. We will start with an organizing month focusing on finances and scheduling the Medical College Admission Test (MCAT).

JANUARY WEEK 1
Money and the MCAT: $$$$$

We start this journey discussing an unmentionable—money. Getting into medical school takes more than top-tier grades, cutting-edge research, and saving-the-world community service. It takes money. The medical school admissions process is obscenely expensive (as is medical school itself), and I want to ensure you have the appropriate amount of cash (or credit or government loans) available before proceeding. Of course, the expense of applying to medical school will vary dramatically depending on the number of schools you apply to and where you interview, but here are some ballpark numbers.

THE PENNY PINCHER ROUTE

ITEM	COST (US $)	COMMENTS
College Transcript Fees	$10	To send transcript to AMCAS
MCAT Books	$100	Used, of course
MCAT Fee	$275	You may apply for the Fee Assistance Program (FAP) to reduce/waive the expense*
AMCAS	$685	Assumes application to 15 schools $160 for one school designation $35 for each school thereafter FAP can reduce/waive the expense
Secondary Applications	$1125	Assumes application to 15 schools Average of $75 each
INTERVIEW TRAVEL		
Gas/Mileage/Bus/ Train/Flight	$500	Assumes 5 interviews
Friend's Couch	$75	For the thank you gift
Food	$75	Breakfast and lunch provided by school You're on your own for dinner
INTERVIEW CLOTHES		
Old Suit/Shirt/Ties	$0	Hope they still fit
New Shoes	$100	More important than you might think
Dry Cleaning	$50	A must
GRAND TOTAL	$2995	

* The Fee Assistance Program (FAP) is provided by the AAMC to applicants whose annual family income is 300% or less of the US Department of Health and Human Services' poverty level guidelines. It can reduce the fee for both the MCAT and AMCAS application. As of 2014, the FAP decreased the MCAT fee from $275 to $100, waived the AMCAS application fee for up to 15 schools, and provided free MCAT and MSAR guides. Visit www.aamc.org/students/applying/fap/ for more details. In addition, many AMCAS-participating medical schools waive their secondary application fees for applicants that receive AAMC-funded FAP.

And that's the cheap route. It also assumes you have excellent independent study habits, friends in every interview location, and a nice suit. Here are more realistic numbers.

THE MORE REALISTIC (AND MORE EXPENSIVE) ROUTE

ITEM	COST (US $)	COMMENTS
MCAT Review Course	$2000	Kaplan and Princeton Review own this market
MCAT Fee	$275	
Admissions Consultant	$325-$5000 (I've used $2500 for calculation)	Offers a huge advantage, particularly regarding strategy, essay editing, and mock interviews
AMCAS	$1035	Assumes application to 25 schools $160 for one school designation $35 for each school thereafter
Secondary Applications	$1875	Assumes application to 25 schools Average of $75 each
INTERVIEW TRAVEL		
Gas/Mileage/Bus/Train/Flight	$1500	Assumes 10 interviews
Hotel/Friend's Couch	$500	Assumes $50/night
Food	$100	
INTERVIEW CLOTHES		
New Suit/Shirt/Ties	$500	
New Shoes	$100	
Dry Cleaning	$50	
GRAND TOTAL	$10535	OUCH

Over $10,000. That is a nice chunk of change. Given that you will likely spend over $200,000 attending medical school (not to mention the opportunity cost of not working during that time), $10,000 is a drop in the bucket. If you want to be a physician, do not let the cost of applying dissuade you. But be an educated consumer and set aside the appropriate amount of savings before you start applying.

JANUARY WEEK 2
Money and the MCAT: Scheduling

Now that we have the distasteful money issue out of the way, let's proceed to an even more unpalatable topic—the Medical College Admission Test (MCAT). Though you may believe standardized testing is a money-making monopoly that does not test your ability to be a doctor, it is a necessary evil. And as much as they hate to admit it, admissions committees pay attention to the score. For those of you with amazing grades, you simply need to show those marks were not a fluke. For those of you who may have faltered in certain classes or are taking a non-traditional path to medical school, the MCAT is your chance to prove you have mastered the required basic science and language skills.

Lucky for you, the MCAT schedule has become more flexible. In the old days (2006 and prior), the MCAT was a written exam only offered twice a year, April and August. This meant almost everyone had to take the exam on one infamous day in April in order to receive his or her scores in time to submit the American Medical College Application Service (AMCAS) application. Now, the MCAT is computer-based and offered on 28 different days spread out over the year. As of 2014, the exam is being offered in January, March, April, May, June, July, August, and September (https://www.aamc.org/students/apply-ing/mcat). With more MCAT dates offered, you can now select a day that maximizes your study time and fits into your overall admissions timeline.

AAMC has started a gold, silver, and bronze zone registration fee structure and policies (https://www.aamc.org/students/download/355350/data/reg-istrationfeesandpolicies.pdf). Registering for the MCAT more than a month prior to the exam puts you into the gold zone and offers cheaper fees and more flexible policies.

As you have likely heard from the pre-med buzz in classrooms and chat rooms, the MCAT is undergoing a large change in 2015. I will review the details of the new exam in the March Year 1: MCAT Prep chapter but want to discuss a few specifics regarding scheduling here. The current (soon to be "old" exam) will be offered through January 2015. If you plan to matriculate to medical school in 2016 or later, you will likely take the new exam, referred to as "MCAT2015." However, pre-meds who have taken the 2014 exam will be able to apply to medical school with the goal of matriculating in 2016 as the

MCAT is valid for three years. When scheduling your exam, please note scores are released about one month after the test date.

As you can expect from any major change, there are many unknowns regarding the MCAT2015. Visit www.aamc.org/mcat for up-to-date information on exam times, registration, and practice tests. And be sure to read the *MCAT Essentials* provided free by AAMC for either test you will be taking. Regardless of the test changes, January is usually the best time to schedule the exam and map out sufficient preparation time.

Here are things to consider when setting your MCAT exam date:

- Will I take a MCAT class or online course?
- When will my class or job schedule allow sufficient study time?
- Will I forget material just learned in classes if I put off taking the exam?
- Will I get my test score back in time to submit the AMCAS application? (AMCAS opens in early June.)
- Will I definitely apply to medical school this cycle? (The MCAT score expires after three years.)
- If I bomb the exam, will I have enough time to retake it? (Be aware that many MCAT sites fill up, and it may be impossible to retake the test unless someone else drops a reservation.)
- Will I be most likely to perform my best on this test date? (You may only take the test three times.)

MEDICAL ADMISSIONS TIMELINE

MCAT
*Year round
*Most take January to May

AMCAS
*Primary application including personal statement and work/activities section
*Opens early May
*Accepts submissions from early June

*Early admissions deadline August 1
*Regular admissions deadlines range from August 1 to December 31

Secondary Applications
*June to February

Interviews
*September to April

Letter of Intent/Update Letters
*Post-interviews
*January to May

JANUARY WEEK 3
Money and the MCAT: Should I Take a MCAT Class?

Whether or not to take a MCAT prep course is often a difficult decision. The answer depends on your economic situation and time management skills. If you have the money and excel in a structured learning environment, a class may be quite helpful. Courses force time management and offer excellent practice tests. But you do not have to take a class to ace the exam. You can easily obtain used study materials and set up a study plan on your own. Also, you can now purchase online review courses that provide increased scheduling flexibility. I passed on a class because I did not have $20 let alone $2000 to spare in college. I bought Kaplan materials from a friend for $50, grudgingly forced myself to study during the summer (I took the August MCAT the year prior to applying), and earned a MCAT score good enough to get me into Harvard. So you can get into medical school without laying out thousands of dollars on a MCAT class. However, I certainly would have taken a class if I had the money. I believe it would have improved my score and dramatically decreased my stress level (no review course paid me to say that, I promise).

Some pre-meds respond better to individualized tutoring than to in-person or online classes. Hiring a private tutor can be an excellent option, particularly if you need help in one specific area. You can find a tutor through test preparation companies, like Kaplan or Princeton Review, or tutoring firms, such as Varsity Tutors (http://www.varsitytutors.com/). But also check out individuals who advertise on campus, in the newspaper, or on Craigslist (www.craigslist.org). The going rate is $150-$200 per hour, but can be cheaper when going through individuals as opposed to large companies.

Here are a few tips to remember when selecting a tutor:

- Focus on hiring a tutor with teaching expertise in your greatest area(s) of need. Earning a high MCAT score does not inherently make someone a strong teacher.
- Shop around. You may have to meet multiple tutors before you find one that clicks.
- Don't be afraid to say it's not working. If the tutor is not producing results or does not mesh with your learning style, find a new one.
- Remember your old teachers. Sometimes high school and college teachers make the best tutors. I have found this to be especially true for the verbal section.

JANUARY WEEK 4
Money and the MCAT: Sign Up

Use this week to sign up for the MCAT. Remember to choose a date that allows sufficient study time and when you definitely will be free from school or work obligations. The 2014 MCAT will be offered on the following dates (check https://www.aamc.org/students/applying/mcat for MCAT2015 dates, due to begin February 2015).

2014 Dates
January 23—8:00 am
January 25—1:00 pm
March 22—1:00 pm
April 5—1:00 pm
April 11—8:00 am
April 24—8:00 am

May 8—1:00 pm
May 17—8:00 am
May 22—8:00 am
May 31—1:00 pm
June 5—1:00 pm
June 13—8:00 am
June 21—8:00 am
July 2—8:00 am
July 12—8:00 am
July 24—1:00 pm
July 25—8:00 am
August 1—8:00 am
August 2—8:00 am
August 7—8:00 am and 2:00 pm
August 15—8:00 am
August 21—1:00 pm
August 27—1:00 pm
September 4—8:00 am
September 6—1:00 pm
September 10—8:00 am and 2:00 pm
September 12—8:00 am
September 18—1:00 pm

2015 Dates (still 2014 MCAT)
January 8—8:00 am
January 10—1:00 pm
January 13—8:00 am

Testing locations can be found at http://services.aamc.org/20/mcat/sitelisting. To officially register and check for updated information, visit the AAMC website at www.aamc.org/students/mcat/start.htm.

The rest of this guide assumes you will take the MCAT the second week of April. If you decide to take it earlier or later, simply shift the schedule provided in this book as needed paying close attention to unchangeable deadlines. Your goal should be to submit the AMCAS in early- to mid-June.

DEADLINES

AMCAS and TMDSAS Early Decision Programs: August 1
AMCAS Regular Decision: August 1-December 31
TMDSAS: October 1
AACOMAS: October 1 to February 1
Secondary deadlines vary by school

If you have decided to take a MCAT course, register now. Two of the most commonly used companies are Kaplan (www.kaptest.com) and Princeton Review (www.princetonreview.com). Of course, these are not the only resources available. A quick Internet search reveals a number of options (because the MCAT is such a money-making enterprise). Other good companies include Examkrackers (www.examkrackers.com) and www.mcat-prep. com. Since the MCAT is now computerized, many students opt for the flexibility of online courses. If you want to go it alone, however, buy MCAT review books now. Check out the following sites for used books:

- Your college's pre-med group or textbook swap system
- www.craigslist.org
- www.half.com/textbooks
- www.campusbooks.com
- www.mcat-bookstore.com
- www.dormitem.com
- www.amazon.com
- www.barnesandnoble.com
- www.ebay.com

CHECKLIST

❑ Arrange for medical school application financing

❑ Sign up for the MCAT

❑ Sign up for a MCAT class/tutor (if you have decided to use one)

❑ Obtain MCAT study materials

NOTES

February Year 1

Recommendations

*"Success always comes when
preparation meets opportunity."*
-HENRY HARTMAN

Think of recommendations, or letters of evaluation as AMCAS likes to call them, as a way for the admissions committee to find out what you are *really* like. But remember that can go both ways. Recommendations are notorious for making or breaking an application. They are an excellent way to show you are well rounded. But one lukewarm or (cringe) outright negative recommendation can sink your chances of becoming a doctor. Now that I've scared you into taking recommendations seriously, let's go over the specifics.

FEBRUARY WEEK 1
Recommendations: How Many?

Most schools require at least three recommendations. I suggest obtaining at least five and then choosing the three you believe will be best for your application to each specific school. Send more than three letters if the school allows it, and if you are confident all the recommendations are strong. It is common to send different numbers of recommendations to different schools given that each school has its own rules. It is always better to send fewer strong recommendations than more mediocre ones. It only takes one lukewarm letter to tarnish an application. Rarely should sending more than five recommendations be necessary. If you plan to send more than five letters, first run the plan by your pre-med committee or an admissions consultant.

If your college writes a composite or pre-med committee letter, then you will like only send this letter. More on such committee letters in February Week 2.

FEBRUARY WEEK 2
Recommendations: Whom Should I Ask?

In general, you should obtain one recommendation from a science teacher, one from a humanities teacher, and one from an extracurricular supervisor. In this way, you can prove your excellence in science, liberal arts, and non-academic endeavors. The goal is to show you are well rounded.

Please, please, please promise me you will focus on obtaining letters of evaluation from individuals who know you well as opposed to big-name professors whom you have never met. A glowing recommendation from your advanced biology teaching assistant whose office hours you visited weekly will be much stronger than a two-line letter from your dad's famous researcher friend whom you met once at the mall. Trust me on this one. I have read hundreds of them. Coaches, community service leaders, and principal investigators may make excellent recommenders. One trick in obtaining recommendations is to ask a teaching assistant or post-bac in the lab who knows you well to write the letter, and then have the professor or principal investigator co-sign the same letter.

Some schools require two science recommendations. Others (such as Harvard) now require a recommendation from every research supervisor listed on your AMCAS work/activities section. Check with each school for specific policies. Also, some schools do not count math as a science. The Texas schools can be particularly picky about such things. Again, check with each school. It never hurts to ask and most schools clearly list their recommendation policies on the admissions website page.

Many schools request a pre-med committee or advisor letter of recommendation from your undergraduate institution. Committee letters fall into three general categories:

1. Pre-Med Committee Composite Letter—Pre-med committee writes a letter composed of excerpts from the letters you already obtained. This is often the only letter sent.
2. Pre-Med Committee Advisor Letter—A unique letter written by the pre-med advisor that is sent along with your other full letters.
3. Letter Packet—The school pre-med committee takes responsibility for sending each full letter you have obtained in one packet. The committee does not write a unique letter.

Be sure to ask your school's pre-med committee if it provides such a letter and how you go about obtaining one. In general, if your school provides a pre-med committee letter and you meet the criteria for obtaining one, the medical school admissions committees want to see the letter regardless of your undergraduate course of study. Even if you are many years out of college or do not like your advisor, applying without a committee letter from a school that provides one is a red flag for admissions committees.

FEBRUARY WEEK 3
Recommendations: How Do I Ask?

Very carefully. Now I don't want you to get nervous when asking for a recommendation, but I do want you to be prepared. First, it's best to start gathering recommendations early. Even if you are a freshman in college, it is not too soon to ask for letters of evaluation. Approach a possible recommender right after you have finished the class (or project or community service) so you are still fresh in his or her mind. You may simply ask that a general recommendation for graduate school be written. This letter can be easily edited into a medical school recommendation at a later date. Here's a step-by-step approach to asking for a letter of evaluation.

1. Set up a face-to face meeting
   Call or e-mail the prospective recommender and ask for a meeting to discuss writing a recommendation. If you cannot arrange a face-to-face meeting, suggest using video conferencing programs, such as Skype,

Facetime, or Google Hangout. If that does not work, request a phone meeting. Do *not* ask for a letter over e-mail because you need to be able to read the face and body language of the potential recommender.

2. Bring the following paperwork for the recommender:
   - Updated curriculum vitae (that's a "CV" or résumé).
   - Transcript (from college, post-baccalaureate, or graduate school; copy is fine).
   - Personal statement (if complete).
   - Recommendation deadline (make it at least three weeks before the published deadline).
   - Pre-addressed, stamped postcard with a statement such as, "I turned in your letter of evaluation to AMCAS today. Good luck. —Dr. Miller." The recommender can drop this postcard in the mail to easily let you know when the recommendation has been submitted.
   - Three items you want the recommender to highlight in the letter.
   - Detailed information about submitting the recommendation, such as the AMCAS Letter Request Form. (See February Week 4 for details.)

3. Ask for a *strong* recommendation
   I mean this literally. During the meeting, ask the recommender point blank if he or she will be able to write a strong letter. If you are squeamish about this, here are some examples of appropriate ways to ask:
   - "Professor Peters, I have enjoyed your class and believe I have excelled in it. I plan to apply to medical school in the future and am hoping you can write me a very strong recommendation. Do you think this would be possible?"
   - "Coach Craig, as you know I am applying to medical school. I think a strong letter from you would help show I have been able to balance both academics and athletics at a high level. Could you write me a strong letter?"
   - "Dr. Dannenberg, I am hoping you will write me a recommendation to medical school detailing my work in your lab and discussing our

upcoming publication. Do you think you can write me a strong recommendation?"

 If the prospective recommender even so much as hesitates in the answer, say thank you for being honest and that you are happy to ask others.

Many college professors write so many recommendations that they use a template and often create a cookie-cutter, bland letter. You may assist the recommender by providing three items to highlight, such as unique experiences, accomplishments, and awards. You can take this strategy one step further and provide three personal qualities backed up with experiences that vary by recommender. This way, you are helping each letter writer show your well-roundedness. Don't be shy about making suggestions. You are actually helping the recommender tremendously by brainstorming what they write about to make your letter stand out.

4. Thanks and follow-up
Once you have heard a resounding, "Yes, it would be my pleasure to write you a strong recommendation for medical school," be sure to give appropriate thanks. Obtain updated contact information (phone, e-mail, mail address) from the recommender so you can check in as the deadline nears or if the deadline is missed (it happens much more often than you'd like to think). I suggest sending a thank you note on the deadline date even if you have not received the self-addressed postcard in the mail. This will act as a memory trigger if your recommender has forgotten the deadline. But if the deadline is missed, no worries. You have already given a deadline three weeks prior to the published date. Aren't you so smart?

Send a second thank you note once you have received admissions to medical schools. You can discuss where you applied, where you gained admissions, and where you are attending. Recommenders love getting the follow-up as so few students take the time to do so. A small gift may be appropriate but is not necessary.

FEBRUARY WEEK 4
Recommendations: Waiver and How to Send

I am often asked, "Should I waive my right to see the recommendations?" The answer is simple, "Always." Waiving your right gives more weight to the letters.

Hopefully, your college or post-baccalaureate school provides a central collection location for recommendations, and then sends them out for you either as a pre-med committee letter or a letter packet. Ask your college's head pre-med counselor what the school provides. If no centralized clearinghouse is available, the recommenders will have to send the recommendations themselves and you are responsible for helping them through the process. There are now various options for this:

1. AMCAS Letter Writer Application

   AMCAS now provides the Letter Writer Application, which allows recommenders to upload the recommendation directly to a website. To use this system, the recommender needs your AAMC ID and Letter ID found on the AMCAS Letter Request Form. This form is downloadable from within the AMCAS application. The Letter Writer Application requires the letter to be saved as a .pdf document. Be sure your recommenders have the software and know how to perform this task. AMCAS provides both insights on what medical school are looking for in letters of evaluation ("https://www.aamc. org/initiatives/admissionsinitiative/332572/lettersofevaluation guidelines.html) and instructions for how to upload letters (https:// www.aamc.org/students/advisors/amcas-advisors/amcas-letters/). I suggest providing both of these website links for your recommenders. The actual Letter Writer Application is https://services.aamc.org/ letterwriter. There is no extra cost for using the Letter Writer Application.

2. Interfolio

   Interfolio is a pay service that can handle your recommendation needs. A one-year subscription costs $19 and each letter sent costs $4-6. A specific AMCAS designation exists within Interfolio. If you choose to use Interfolio or your university requires you do so, you can give recommenders this link: http://www.interfolio.com/recommendationwriters/index.cfm. It explains how letters can be either uploaded or mailed.

3. VirtualEvals

Many schools that write pre-med committee letters use VirtualEvals, which is available to members of the National Association of Advisors for the Health Professions. If your school uses VirtualEvals, you will give the AMCAS Letter Request Form to whomever is writing the committee letter, along with an envelope stamped and addressed to your pre-med committee. The pre-med committee will then send in the recommendation through VirtualEvals (http://www.virtualevals.org/).

4. US Mail

If your school does not compile recommendations for you, traditional mail is another option. In addition, some recommenders prefer old school methods of submitting recommendations. If so, the recommendation along with the Letter Request Form should be sent to:

> AMCAS, attn: AMCAS Letters
> AAMC Medical School Application Services
> P.O. Box 18958
> Washington, DC 20036

When using this method, be sure to provide the recommender with the Letter Request Form and a pre-addressed, stamped envelope.

Please note some schools will not accept letters of recommendation through AMCAS. The list of schools accepting AMCAS recommendations can be found here: http://www.aamc.org/students/amcas/faq/amcasletters.htm.

The AAMC has created an excellent AMCAS letters of recommendation frequently asked question page that is a must read prior to asking for recommendations: http://www.aamc.org/students/applying/amcas/faqs/146562/letters_questions_landing_page.html.

CHECKLIST

❑ Determine whom to ask for recommendations

❑ Gather recommendation packet materials to give to each recommender

❑ Ask for strong recommendations

NOTES

March Year 1

MCAT Prep

"Every worthwhile accomplishment, big or little, has its stages of drudgery and triumph; a beginning, a struggle, and a victory."
-MOHANDAS GANDHI

Perhaps you couldn't come up with the money for a MCAT course or decided that you are wicked smart and disciplined. Either way, these next chapters assume you are going to study for the MCAT on your own. If you are taking the test the second week of April, it is time to hit the books. Please note that if you are working full time and have not taken a science class in five years, you will likely need to dedicate more than five weeks to studying. Please take these chapters as a simple, general guideline to MCAT preparation.

To give you a sense of the amount of time you need to put in, a typical private course provides 18 three-hour classroom sessions, eight AAMC computerized exams, an additional 11 full-length computerized exams, 10,000 practice items, and 1,300 pages of study material plus flashcards. Believe me, I am not proposing you take a course (I didn't). I just want you to have a sense of the huge amount of time you will need to study and master all this material.

Given all of the recent and future changes to the MCAT, let's start with an overview of the test. If you plan to take MCAT2015, feel free to skip over the 2014 test discussion.

2014 MCAT: As of 2013, the AAMC create a MCAT exam to be administered through January 2015 and only consisting of three official sections. The writing sample has been removed and replaced with a voluntary trial section to test questions for the new MCAT2015 exam. Those who participate in the trial section receive a $30 Amazon gift card. Given 2013 is now behind us, the AAMC is now referring to this test as the 2014 MCAT. It has four parts:

- Physical Sciences (PS)
- Verbal Reasoning (VR)
- Biological Sciences (BS)
- Trial Section (TS)

IMPORTANT 2014 MCAT FACTS

- The test is a little over five hours long including breaks.
- Total content time is approximately four hours and five minutes.
- The test is self-paced (i.e., you choose when to take a break) but each section has a time limit.
- You are able to review and change answers within a section until you reach the time limit for that particular section. Unfortunately, once you have completed a section, you cannot go back and change answers.
- You may make notations on the screen such as highlighting a passage or striking out an answer choice.
- Scores will be available in approximately 30 days after exam completion. Scores are sent directly to AMCAS. Be sure to select sending scores to your pre-med advisor as well (it's free).
- If you think you performed very poorly on the exam, you can cancel the score at the end of the test and it will be voided. There is no way to cancel the score once you leave the exam site.
- You may only take the MCAT three times in one year. Voided exams and "no shows" count as one of your three attempts.
- Only one MCAT reservation may be held at any one time.
- MCAT scores expire in three years.

Here's a breakdown of the test sections, questions, and time limits from the AAMC's *MCAT Essentials* for 2014 and January 2015, a free publication available as a pdf document at https://www.aamc.org/students/download/63060/data/mcatessentials.pdf.

TEST SECTION	QUESTIONS	TIME
Name Confirmation Screen		2 minutes
Examinee Agreement		10 minutes
Tutorial (optional)		10 minutes
Physical Sciences	52	70 minutes
Break (optional)		10 minutes
Verbal Reasoning	40	60 minutes
Break (optional)		10 minutes
Biological Sciences	52	70 minutes
Void Question		5 minutes
Break (optional)		10 minutes
Trial Section (optional)	32	45 minutes
Satisfaction Survey (optional)	12	10 minutes
Total Content Time		4 hours, 5 minutes
Total Seat Time		5 hours, 10 minutes

The PS, VR, and BS sections are scored on a scale of 15 (15 being the highest score possible). The trial section is not scored.

You will see scores reported as:

PS 15 VR 15 BS 15 or 45

MCAT2015: This new test is due to begin in February 2015 and will affect pre-meds applying for entry to medical school in 2016 and later. The AAMC spent three years studying how to improve the MCAT to better reflect recent advances in medical science and the need for "softer" skills to excel as a physician. They have created a comprehensive, 158-page *Preview Guide for the MCAT2015 Exam* available for free download at https://www.aamc.org/students/applying/mcat/. This document covers every detail of the MCAT change including sample questions.

SUMMARY OF 2015 MCAT CHANGES

- Biological sciences section is now called, "Biological and Biochemical Foundations of Living Systems."
- Physical sciences section is now called, "Chemical and Physical Foundations of Biological Systems."

    Both of these sections, referred to collectively as the "natural sciences" will continue to test concepts in biology, general and organic chemistry, biochemistry, and physics and will be updated to reflect the information medical school faculty believe is most important for success in medical school.

• Addition of a new social and behavioral science section called, "Psychological, Social, and Biological Foundations of Behavior."

This section will test knowledge of introductory psychiatry and sociology, in addition to biological concepts relating to mental process and behavior. Understanding of basic research methods and statistics will also be tested.

• Verbal reasoning section is now called, "Critical Analysis and Reasoning Skills."

This section requires analysis and application of information provided in passages from social science and humanities disciplines. Passages will include subjects such as ethics, philosophy, cross-cultural studies, and population health. Similar to the previous verbal reasoning section, you may be asked to decipher the tone and overall view of the passage author.

Just like the current physical sciences, verbal reasoning, and biological sciences sections, the MCAT2015's four sections will be scored on a 1-15 scale. Four sections, four scores.

The expected breakdown of the test sections, questions, and time limits is as follows:

TEST SECTION	QUESTIONS	TIME
Biological and Biochemical Foundations of Living Systems	67	95 minutes
Chemical and Physical Foundations of Biological Systems	67	95 minutes
Psychological, Social, and Biological Foundations of Behavior	67	95 minutes
Critical Analysis and Reasoning Skills	60	90 minutes

The AAMC will continue to offer low-cost test preparation materials. On the AAMC MCAT2015 website (https://www.aamc.org/students/applying/

mcat/mcat2015/), you can find an informational video featuring advice on how to prepare for the new exam. In 2014, a full-length practice test will be posted on the site allowing pre-meds to simulate the actual test, and *The Official Guide to MCAT2015* will be released. Further, in 2015, the AAMC will release a second full-length practice exam.

As with all new standardized exams, there will be considerable anxiety from both pre-meds and admissions committees regarding how to interpret the scores. While the AAMC works out the kinks and test preparation companies determine how best to prepare pre-meds for the exam, it is possible the MCAT will carry slightly less weight than usual. But certainly don't count on it!

Regardless of which exam you take, you likely want to know what score is required to gain admission. Data compiled by the AAMC shows that no MCAT score guarantees admissions to medical school. However, applications scores in each section of >10 are more likely to be accepted. We can only assume this trend will continue with the MCAT2015.

When preparing for any MCAT exam, have the mindset that you will only sit the test once. You should never go into the MCAT unprepared as a "practice" session because medical schools see every unexpired score.

Many applicants wonder if they should retake the MCAT. Generally speaking, you should only retest if you can improve your score by at least three points (which is quite hard to do). Good reasons for retaking the test include:

- You simply were not prepared (did not study well, had not taken the appropriate classes).
- You were sick as a dog on test day.
- You freaked out.
- Your score is very uneven and you strongly believe you can improve the low score (for example, PS 7 VR 11 BS 12 and you are confident you can improve the PS to 10).
- Your score is less than 30 and you strongly believe you can get it above 30 (ideally three or more points higher).

Remember, unless you cancelled your score at the end of the test, the admissions committees will see every MCAT score you have earned that has not expired. MCAT scores expire after three years and you may take the test only three times in a given year.

The AAMC did a survey of medical school admissions committees to see how they use multiple MCAT scores. The survey revealed several methods. Some schools view all scores equally and look for improvement. Others look only at the most recent score. Some average all scores. Still others take the highest score. Of these four methods, the first is most common.

MCAT STUDY TIPS

- Don't waste time studying things you already know. Mastered Van der Waal's forces and Zeroth's law? Why study them again? Many students fall into the trap of reviewing what they know to boost confidence. If you take this tactic, you may not have enough time to master what you don't know. What's the point of studying if you aren't going to learn anything new?
- Answers with extremes such as "always" and "never" are rarely correct.
- If two answers are very similar, one is likely to be the right answer.
- Eliminate any answers you know are wrong immediately. This will often leave you with two answers to decide between (and a 50/50 shot at answering correctly).
- If you think of an answer before you see the list and that answer is present, it is likely to be correct.

MARCH WEEK 1
MCAT Prep: Verbal Reasoning
(Critical Analysis and Reasoning Skills for MCAT2015)

I suggest beginning your MCAT studying with the verbal reasoning/critical analysis and reasoning skills (VR/CARS) section because it is often the most difficult for pre-meds. Why it is so hard? Two main reasons: most pre-meds have left side of the brain tendencies and language/reading comprehension skills cannot be mastered overnight. Despite it's non-science subject, the VR/CARS score is just as important as the science section scores because data shows a pre-med's performance on this MCAT section directly correlates with his or her United States Medical Licensing Examination (USMLE) Step 1 board score taken in medical school. Medical schools care very much about your likelihood of passing the USMLE as the schools are often judged by their students' pass rate.

Certain techniques can be learned and generally lead to a higher score. The key is practice. Remember, no factual knowledge is tested. The purpose is to evaluate your reasoning and critical thinking ability.

This week you should read the verbal reasoning/critical analysis and reasoning skills section of your review books and then do as many practice tests as physically possible on the computer. Hopefully, your review books include practice tests via DVD or online" after "practice tests. The more questions you complete, the more patterns you will see. Time is often a factor in this section, so be sure to time yourself and become accustomed to reading quickly and accurately on a computer screen.

There are several different strategies for how to approach the VR/CARS section. Here are some examples:

- Read the entire passage quickly to obtain the overall tone and argument → read the questions and answer any you can → return to the passage looking for the details necessary to answer the remaining questions.
- Read the questions first → read the passage → answer the questions.
- Read the passage deliberately focusing on both overarching argument and details → answer the questions.

I can't predict which strategy will work best for you. Try each on a practice test and see which one you like best. Then use that strategy over and over on practice tests until it becomes second nature.

Though your MCAT review book will go over many verbal reasoning test-taking strategies, here are a few specifics I think are most important:

- The VR/CARS section focuses on the overall argument and tone of the passage and not the details. This is very different from what you learn in a typical science class. The key is to distinguish fact from opinion. Read the passage as if you are debating with the author. Focus on the author's tone, style, supporting evidence, and any holes in thinking you could attack in a debate. Pay attention to words implying an author's view or opinion such as additionally, but, further, however, in contrast, nevertheless, then, therefore, thus, primarily, and yet. Remember, you don't have to understand every detail of an abstract passage to understand the overall argument.

- Don't waste tons of time annotating the passage. Never write full sentences. Just jot down little notes. Shorthand and abbreviations work well. No one has to understand the annotations but you. Time is often a huge factor in the VR/CARS test, so use it wisely.
- Inference questions can be a beast. If a question is asking you to infer something from the passage, remember the true answer *must* be true based on the passage. If there is any doubt (*i.e.*, the answer *may* not be true) then it is not the correct answer.
- Try to predict the answer before looking at the options. If what is in your head is an answer, it is probably right.
- Do not bring outside knowledge into your VR/CARS answers. Everything you need to answer the questions exists within the passage.

MARCH WEEK 2
MCAT Prep: Physical Sciences
(Chemical and Physical Foundations of
Biological Systems for MCAT2015)

The physical sciences/chemical and physical foundations of biological systems (PS/CPF) portion of the MCAT tests chemistry and physics, with both physical and organic chemistry as fair game. However, if you loved orgo as much as I did (ok, it was the most painful class I have ever taken), don't despair. Basic organic chemistry knowledge should be sufficient. The physics knowledge tested does not require calculus.

This week, read the chemistry and physics portions of your review book once. Then take the physical sciences practice tests. Mark the incorrect answers and then review only those sections relevant to the questions you missed. Don't waste time re-reading things you already know. It may make you feel good to see familiar facts and formulas, but reviewing the subjects you have already mastered is throwing time and energy out the window. Focus on what you don't know.

MARCH WEEK 3
MCAT Prep: Social Sciences
(Psychological, Social, and Biological Foundations
of Behavior for MCAT2015)

Despite all the fancy name changes, psychological, social, and biological foundations of behavior (PSB) is really the only markedly new addition to MCAT2015. If you are taking the 2014 MCAT, use this week to re-review verbal reasoning or get a head start on biological sciences. If you plan to take MCAT2015, read on.

The AAMC added PSB to MCAT 2015 in an effort to highlight the importance of social sciences, such as psychiatry and sociology, in medicine. Statistics and research methods will also be tested. As no one but the test makers know exactly what will be covered, you should rely heavily on the information and practice tests provided on the AAMC MCAT2015 website.

This week, review the AAMC MCAT 2015 guides and practice tests focusing on the PSB information and questions. Then turn to your MCAT prep books, reading the PSB section and taking any practice tests provided. Review only the questions you have missed.

MARCH WEEK 4
MCAT Prep: Biological Sciences
(Biological and Biochemical Foundations
of Living Systems for MCAT2015)

Most students applying to medical school find biology the most intuitive of all science subjects. The MCAT writers know this and often make the biological sciences/biological and biochemical foundations of living systems (BS/BBF) section harder than you would expect in order to create a spread in the scores. They certainly don't want everyone to score a 15. Since biology involves a significant amount of memorization, I suggest you study this subject last so the facts are fresh in your mind on test day.

Read the BS/BBF sections of your review book this week. Then take the BS/BBF practice tests. Review only those sections you have missed.

CHECKLIST

❑ Review MCAT format

❑ Study all four sections (Three for 2014 MCAT test takers)

❑ Take practice tests from each section and review questions missed

NOTES

April Year 1
Final MCAT Prep, CV, and Transcripts

"Just go out there and do what you've got to do."
- Martina Navratilova

It's April. Flowers are blooming and spring is in the air. It's beautiful outside and you are locked in your room studying. Never fear, freedom is near. At least freedom from studying for the MCAT. The first part of April is dedicated to the MCAT. Once you celebrate finishing the exam, preparing for the AMCAS application will begin.

APRIL WEEK 1
MCAT Prep: Practice Tests

Spend this week taking full timed tests. Full-length practice tests can be found at www.aamc.org/mcat. You hopefully obtained other full-length tests along with your study materials. Grade each test then immediately review the subject areas of the questions you missed. Repeat. Take as many full tests as you can. Remember to time yourself every time. Many people underperform on the MCAT only because they run out of time.

APRIL WEEK 2
MCAT: Showtime!

It's the week of the test. Spend the beginning of the week reviewing last minute facts. Yes, it is time to cram. All those silly details (insert "Kreb's Cycle" here) you will likely never need in real life should be mashed, jammed, and wrestled into your head now. Many MCAT books have a rapid review section perfect for this purpose.

Two nights before the test, get a full eight hours of sleep. Sleep experts have shown that the "night before the night before" is the most critical night of sleep to ensure highest performance on exams.

The day before the test do *not* study. Yes, I said don't study. You have done enough already and one day is not going to make or break you. Take the day off and try to relax. Go to dinner and a movie. Rest your mind. Don't even peek at those review books.

The night before the test, review how to get to the exam site, pack snacks and a bag lunch, and get to sleep early.

The morning of the test, stay with your usual morning routine. Before leaving home, ensure you have a valid ID containing both a signature and photo (passport or driver's license). An expired ID will not be considered valid. Wear layers in case the test center is hotter or colder than you like. Arrive at the test center 30 minutes before your appointment time. A locker will be provided to store your personal items. Unfortunately, you will not be able to choose your computer. Noise-reducing headsets/earplugs will be made available by the test center to help you concentrate.

Take the MCAT and celebrate.

APRIL WEEK 3
Review CV

Once you have celebrated finishing one of the hardest exams you will ever take, it is time to start thinking about actually applying to medical school. To help prepare for filling out the AMCAS application, dust off that old CV (the one you handed to recommenders in February). Updating your CV now will make completing the AMCAS application much simpler. Pre-med CVs usually include sections on education, work experience, community service/volunteerism, extracurriculars/sports/arts/clubs, research/publications, clinical experience, skills, and hobbies. Each experience you mention should be associated with a time, place, and brief explanation. Think back over your academic and work career and brainstorm what experiences meant the most to your growth as a student and as a person. Research exact experience dates and names of supervisors you may have forgotten. At this stage, it is best to write down every experience you think might be included in the AMCAS. You will flesh out exactly what to put on the application in May.

APRIL WEEK 4
Obtain Transcripts

Did you know you can request transcripts to be sent to AMCAS even before your application is complete?

Medical schools require transcripts from every post-secondary school you have attended. This includes all junior colleges, community colleges, trade schools, or graduate schools. You have to submit a transcript even if no credit was earned from a course.

AMCAS provides a transcript request form within the application. Even though you can't fill out, print, and submit the transcript request form until the AMCAS application opens on May 1, you can order an unofficial transcript from each post-secondary school. Do this now, as you will need the transcripts in order to fill out the "Schools Attended" section of the application. Though many universities give you immediate access to your unofficial transcript online, some require you to submit a formal request and pay a fee. Then, you often have to wait weeks to receive access to the transcript or have it e-mailed/ mailed to you. By researching how to obtain an unofficial transcript this week, you will be ready to submit the official transcript request form when AMCAS opens May 1 and to start filling out the AMCAS Schools Attended section in the coming weeks.

The transcript deadline for the AMCAS Early Decision Program is August 1. For regular applications, the deadline is at 5pm Eastern Standard Time (EST) 14 calendar days after a particular school's stated application deadline. If the transcript deadline is a weekend or holiday, materials are due the following business day. But these deadlines won't be an issue for you because you will submit a transcript request form to the office of registrar of every post-secondary school attended on May 1. See May Week 1 for more details.

CHECKLIST

❑ Take full timed MCAT practice tests

❑ Ace the MCAT

❑ Review and update CV

❑ Obtain unofficial transcripts from each post-secondary school attended

NOTES

May Year 1

AMCAS Application

"Put it before them briefly so they will read it, clearly so they will appreciate it, picturesquely so they will remember it, and above all, accurately so they will be guided by its light."
-JOSEPH PULITZER

Now the actual applying begins. The American Medical College Application Service (AMCAS) is a centralized application processing service for those applying to allopathic medical schools in the United States. AMCAS has nothing to do with the admissions decisions—that's the job of each school's individual admissions committee. The vast majority of medical schools use this service. But in true Texas style, some schools in that state use another system called Texas Medical and Dental Schools Application Service (TMDSAS). To make it even more confusing, you apply to some Texas schools' MD/PhD programs through AMCAS. If you are applying to schools in the Great State of Texas, be sure to check early to determine which application processing service to use. For the most up-to-date information on AMCAS-participating schools, visit www.aamc.org/students/applying/amcas/participating_schools/. If you are applying to DO or Canadian schools, separate application services exist. One of the best resources for determining which schools accept which service is the *Medical School Admission Requirements* (MSAR) which can be purchased at https://www.aamc.org/students/applying/requirements/msar/ for $12–22 depending on format. AMCAS usually begins accepting applications in the first week of June.

IMPORTANT APPLICATION WEBSITES

AMCAS: www.aamc.org/amcas

TMDSAS: http://www.utsystem.edu/tmdsas/

OMSAS: http://www.ouac.on.ca/omsas/ (rest of Canadian schools have
individual applications)

AACOMAS: http://aacomas.aacom.org/

OTHER HELPFUL WEBSITES

AAMC: www.aamc.org

Main source of information for MD applicants

AACOM: www.aacom.org

Best resource for DO applicants

The Student Doctor Network: www.studentdoctor.net

Free subscription service providing forums for medical types of
all levels (pre-med, pre-dental, veterinary medicine, pharmacy,
residency, *etc.*)

Old Premeds: www.oldpremeds.org

For non-traditional pre-med candidates

MomMD: www.mommd.com

Resource for women in medicine

MAY WEEK 1
AMCAS: Sections I-IV, VI, VII, and IX

The AMCAS application (www.aamc.org/amcas), often referred to as the "primary" application, opens May 1. Though you can't submit the application until early June, you may and should start working on it. These coming weeks will focus on the AMCAS, but you can follow the same basic timeline if you are applying to TMDSAS and/or AACOMAS.

Dedicate this week to completing administrative-heavy tasks. "AMCAS: Sections I-IV, VI, VII, and IX" sounds like a lot of work, doesn't it? Fortunately, the effort you have put in during previous weeks will make these tasks much easier.

Here are the specifics on what you can fill out this week:

I. Identifying Information

Enter your name, birth information, and sex. If only the whole application was this easy.

II. Schools Attended

In this section, you will provide information on all of the post-high school educational institutions you have attended. This includes community college, summer school, and study abroad programs. You will also be asked about previous matriculation into medical school and any institutional action filed against you.

Medical schools take institutional action very seriously. The worst thing you can do is withhold information and have the medical school admissions committees find out about an incident later – this will undoubtedly lead to a rejection even if you have already been accepted into medical school. As stated on the AMCAS webpage, any "academic performance or a conduct violation, even if such action did not interrupt your enrollment, require you to withdraw, or does not appear on your official transcripts due to institutional policy or personal petition" must be acknowledged and explained. When writing about such experiences, it is best to be brief. In 1325 characters or less, describe what happened and what you learned from it. Admissions committees do not want to read lengthy sob stories. I have seen many applicants thwarted by institutional action regarding illegal use of alcohol while underage. Hopefully knowing the strictness of AMCAS' rules will be added incentive for you to make good decisions.

Once you have completed AMCAS sections I and II, you may request official transcripts by printing out and submitting the transcript request form to your registrar(s).

III. Biographic Information

AMCAS section III requests your biographic information, such as address, phone number, e-mail, citizenship, legal residence, languages spoken, race/ethnicity, childhood and family information, military service, and any misdemeanor or felony charges. Though this should be an easy section to complete, many pre-meds struggle with it. A few things to note:

- AMCAS communicates mainly via e-mail, so be sure to input a valid e-mail address you will check regularly for the next year(s).
- Legal residence is of great import, as it affects where you are considered an "in-state applicant." If your legal residency is unclear, do some research on the residency rules of each state in question. These rules may often be found on state-run websites and usually include elements such as where you pay taxes, own/rent property, pay utilities, and are registered to vote.
- The race/ethnicity questions often cause great angst for many applicants. The key is to be honest. And if you don't want to answer the questions, you don't have to. They are optional.
- AMCAS asks many personal questions about your family background in an attempt to determine your "disadvantaged" status, including parents'/guardians' level of education and current employment information, number and age of siblings, family's income, and details about how you paid for college. These questions stem from many medical schools trying to move their affirmative action policies away from assessing race and ethnicity to a more comprehensive evaluation of a candidate's access to opportunities. If you come from a disadvantaged background, do not be ashamed to admit it. "Disadvantaged" does not refer only to racial or ethnic status because the economic, familial, and geographic details of your upbringing may also play a role. Medical school admissions committees take disadvantaged status very seriously and often give applicants who have overcome barriers an advantage in the application process. AMCAS requests applicants with are potentially disadvantaged to answer the question, "Do you believe you have faced any hardships from birth to present that interfered with your educational pursuits?" If you are unsure whether or not you meet disadvantaged status criteria, speak with your college's premed advisor or a medical school admissions consultant who can help guide you.
- This section also requests you disclose and explain any misdemeanors or felonies.
- In addition to asking about misdemeanor and felony charges, the AMCAS application also states that if you "are convicted of, plead guilty, or no contest to a felony or misdemeanor crime, you must

inform the admissions office of each medical school to which you have applied" if the event occurs after the submissions date. I know of multiple pre-meds accepted into medical school and then convicted of driving while under the influence of alcohol or possession of illicit substances. Every medical school subsequently withdrew acceptances. Even after you press the AMCAS submission button or receive a letter of acceptance, you are still obligated to be a law-abiding citizen.

IV. Coursework

This is where your transcript(s) will be essential. For every school you have attended, enter academic status, course number, course name, course classification, course type, credit hours, and official transcript grade. Once you have input the data, the AMCAS system will automatically generate your GPA and break it down into:

- Cumulative GPA
- Science GPA (i.e., BCPM – biology, chemistry, physics, and math)
- All Other GPA (AO)

Remember, you have to enter every course taken after high school, even if no credit was earned. AMCAS even wants to see "courses removed from your transcripts or GPA as a result of academic bankruptcy, forgiveness, or similar institutional policies." They are tough! The only courses that do not count towards to AMCAS GPA are pass/fail – pass, pass/fail – fail, advanced placement (AP) credit, College Level Examination Program (CLEP) credit, audited courses, and courses officially withdrawn or "dropped." AMCAS reports the total hours for these first four types of courses under a "Supplementary Hours" heading.

AMCAS verifies every course based on your official transcript and calculates GPAs prior to transmitting applications to medical schools. Of note, AMCAS often generates different GPAs than many undergraduate institutions because it counts virtually every course and has a standard calculation for "+" and "-" grades. In general, AMCAS GPAs are a tad lower than transcript grades. Rarely have I seen a GPA change by more than one tenth unless AMCAS counts a course with a poor grade that a pre-med's university did not.

Here is an example of how AMCAS presents grades to medical schools:

STATUS	BCPM		AO		TOTAL	
	GPA	HOURS	GPA	HOURS	GPA	HOURS
High School						
Freshman	3.47	17.00	2.75	12.00	3.17	29.00
Sophomore	3.32	19.00	4.00	18.00	3.65	37.00
Junior	3.77	22.00	4.00	6.00	3.82	28.00
Senior	3.75	24.00			3.75	24.00
Postbaccalaureate Undergraduate						
Cumulative Undergraduate	3.6	82.00	3.58	36.00	3.59	118.00
Graduate	4.00	4.00			4.00	4.00
Supplemental Hours	P/F – PASS: 2.00	P/F – FAIL:	A/P: 39.00	CLEP:	OTHER: 2.00	

Entering course classification and study abroad classes often causes confusion for applicants. Between AAMC's *Course Classification Guide* (https://www.aamc.org/students/download/181694/data/amcas_ course_classification_guide.pdf) and *AMCAS Instruction Manual* (https://www.aamc.org/students/download/182162/data/amcas_ instruction_manual.pdf), you will be able to find out the answers to even your most esoteric course classification questions. Don't just guess on how to classify courses, as it could lead to a delay in your AMCAS application being certified. Remember, someone at AMCAS checks every course and grade to ensure you entered it properly. When in doubt, look it up or call/e-mail the AAMC.

V. Work/Activities

May Week 2 is dedicated to the AMCAS Work/Activities section, so we'll skip it for now.

VI. Letters of Evaluation

Fortunately, you already organized recommendation letters in February. Enter the names and contact information of all recommenders in this section.

VII. Medical Schools

Before entering your school list in AMCAS, you need to decide which general program you will follow. Do you want to be an MD/PhD? How about getting a dual MD/MBA? Or perhaps you know exactly where you want to apply and hope to be accepted early. No matter what path you choose, it will require some research to learn the exact rules and requirements for each track. Here are some general guidelines:

- Early Decision Program (EDP): You may apply to only one school and will find out by October 1 if you are accepted. If you don't get in, you may then turn in a regular AMCAS application. This approach is fantastic if you are a stellar candidate and know exactly where you want to go to school. However, it is risky for most. If you are not accepted, you will be submitting an application much later than the rest of the applicants, a huge detriment when it comes to rolling admissions schools. You are not allowed to apply to the EDP and AMCAS at the same time. The EDP deadline is August 1.

- Regular MD: Follow the AMCAS guidelines. The application deadlines vary by school and range from August to December. Remember some Texas and all DO schools require separate applications.

- MD/PhD: This program is for candidates who want to focus on research. MD/PhD students generally complete their first two years of medical school, head off to lab for three to seven years, and return to complete medical school upon finishing their PhD research. Many are drawn to the MD/PhD path because the school subsidizes tuition. However, money is certainly not a reason to pursue this course. Schools expect you to enter this program because you love research, and you will need to prove a talent for research to the admissions committees. MD/PhD candidates are required to submit two extra essays through AMCAS.

- Other combined programs: Many schools are starting to offer combined programs such as MD/MBA, MD/JD, MD/MPH, and MD/MPA. Such programs often shave a year off of the regular requirements compared to attending each school separately. Joint degree programs are becoming more popular, so be sure to check with each school to see if any such programs exist or will exist in the near future. You will have to contact each school separately for the specific application. Many schools will have you apply to the joint program once accepted into the medical school.

AMCAS-PARTICIPATING SCHOOLS
BY DEADLINES FOR 2014 ENTERING CLASS
(MODIFIED FROM WWW.AAMC.ORG)

AUGUST 1 DEADLINE
University of Missouri Kansas City School of Medicine

AUGUST 31 DEADLINE
University of Michigan Medical School (M.D.-Ph.D.)

SEPTEMBER 30 DEADLINE
University of California, San Diego School of Medicine (MD/PhD)
University of Michigan Medical School (Regular M.D.)

OCTOBER 1 DEADLINE
Mayo Medical School
Texas A&M Health Sciences Center School of Medicine (M.D.-Ph.D.)
Texas Tech University Health Sciences Center School of Medicine
    (M.D.-Ph.D.)
University of California, Davis School of Medicine

OCTOBER 15 DEADLINE
Columbia University College of Physicians and Surgeons
Duke University School of Medicine
Emory University School of Medicine
Harvard Medical School
Icahn School of Medicine at Mount Sinai
Jefferson Medical College of Thomas Jefferson University (M.D.-Ph.D.)

Johns Hopkins University School of Medicine
New York University School of Medicine
Northwestern University Feinberg School of Medicine
Oregon Health and Science University School of Medicine
Raymond and Ruth Perelman School of Medicine at the Univ.
  of Pennsylvania
Sanford School of Medicine of the University of South Dakota (M.D.-Ph.D.)
Stanford University School of Medicine
State University of New York Upstate Medical University College of Medicine
Tulane University School of Medicine (M.D.-Ph.D.)
University of Arizona College of Medicine-Phoenix
University of California, San Francisco School of Medicine
Univ. of Chicago Division of the Biological Sci. The Pritzker School of Medicine
University of Kansas School of Medicine
University of Louisville School of Medicine
University of Mississippi School of Medicine
University of Missouri-Columbia School of Medicine
University of Nevada School of Medicine
University of North Carolina School of Medicine (M.D.-Ph.D.)
University of North Dakota School of Medicine and Health Sciences
University of Oklahoma College of Medicine
University of Pittsburgh School of Medicine
University of Rochester School of Medicine and Dentistry
University of Virginia School of Medicine (M.D.-Ph.D.)
University of Washington School of Medicine
Virginia Commonwealth University School of Medicine
Washington University in St. Louis School of Medicine (M.D.-Ph.D.)
Weill Cornell Medical College
Yale University School of Medicine

NOVEMBER 1 DEADLINE
Albany Medical College
Albert Einstein College of Medicine of Yeshiva University

Baylor College of Medicine

Boston University School of Medicine

Case Western Reserve University School of Medicine

Chicago Medical School at Rosalind Franklin University of Medicine
   and Science

Creighton University School of Medicine

Drexel University College of Medicine (M.D.-Ph.D.)

Geisel School of Medicine at Dartmouth

Georgetown University School of Medicine

Keck School of Medicine of the University of Southern California

Loma Linda University School of Medicine

Louisiana State University Health Sciences Center School of Medicine
   in Shreveport

Marshall University Joan C. Edwards School of Medicine

Medical College of Georgia at Georgia Regents University

Medical College of Wisconsin

Mercer University School of Medicine

Michigan State University College of Human Medicine

Northeast Ohio Medical University College of Medicine

Ohio State University College of Medicine

Rush Medical College of Rush University Medical Center

The University of Toledo College of Medicine

The Warren Alpert Medical School of Brown University

Tufts University School of Medicine

University of Alabama School of Medicine

University of Arizona College of Medicine

University of Arkansas for Medical Sciences College of Medicine

University of California Irvine College of Medicine

University of California Los Angeles David Geffen School of Medicine

University of California San Diego School of Medicine (Regular M.D.)

University of Colorado School of Medicine

University of Hawaii John A. Burns School of Medicine

University of Illinois College of Medicine (Regular M.D.)

University of Iowa Roy J. and Lucille A. Carver College of Medicine
University of Kentucky College of Medicine
University of Maryland School of Medicine
University of Massachusetts Medical School
University of Nebraska Medical Center College of Medicine
University of North Carolina School of Medicine (Regular M.D.)
University of Texas Medical School at Houston (M.D.-Ph.D.)
University of Texas Medical School at San Antonio (M.D.-Ph.D.)
University of Texas Southwestern Medical Center at Dallas
   Southwestern Medical School (M.D.-Ph.D.)
University of Utah School of Medicine
University of Virginia School of Medicine (Regular M.D.)
University of Wisconsin School of Medicine and Public Health
Vanderbilt University School of Medicine
Wake Forest School of Medicine of Wake Forest University Baptist
   Medical Center
Wayne State University School of Medicine (M.D.-Ph.D.)
West Virginia University School of Medicine
Wright State University Boonshoft School of Medicine

NOVEMBER 15 DEADLINE
East Tennessee State University James H. Quillen College of Medicine
Eastern Virginia Medical School
Jefferson Medical College of Thomas Jefferson University (Regular M.D.)
Louisiana State University School of Medicine in New Orleans (M.D.-Ph.D.)
Loyola University Chicago Stritch School of Medicine
Oakland University William Beaumont School of Medicine
Pennsylvania State University College of Medicine
Sanford School of Medicine of the University of South Dakota
   (Regular M.D.)
Southern Illinois University School of Medicine
The Brody School of Medicine at East Carolina University
UCLA/Drew Medical Education Program

Uniformed Services University of the Health Sciences F. Edward Hebert
    School of Medicine
University at Buffalo School of Medicine and Biomedical Sciences,
    State University of New York
University of California, Riverside School of Medicine
University of Cincinnati College of Medicine
University of Connecticut School of Medicine
University of Minnesota Medical School
University of New Mexico School of Medicine
University of South Alabama College of Medicine
University of Tennessee Health Science Center College of Medicine
University of Texas Medical Branch at Galveston (M.D.-Ph.D. only)
University of Vermont College of Medicine
USF Health Morsani College of Medicine
Western Michigan University School of Medicine

NOVEMBER 30 DEADLINE
Central Michigan University College of Medicine
Louisiana State University School of Medicine in New Orleans
    (Regular M.D.)

DECEMBER 1 DEADLINE
Morehouse School of Medicine
State University of New York Downstate Medical Center College
    of Medicine
The Frank H. Netter MD School of Medicine at Quinnipiac University
Washington University in Saint Louis School of Medicine (Regular M.D.)

DECEMBER 2 DEADLINE
Drexel University College of Medicine (Regular M.D.)
Florida State University College of Medicine
George Washington University School of Medicine and Health Sciences
Hofstra North Shore-LIJ School of Medicine

Medical University of South Carolina College of Medicine
Stony Brook University School of Medicine
University of Central Florida College of Medicine
University of Florida College of Medicine
University of Miami Leonard M. Miller School of Medicine
University of Puerto Rico School of Medicine (Regular M.D.)
University of South Carolina School of Medicine
Virginia Tech Carilion School of Medicine

DECEMBER 15 DEADLINE
Saint Louis University School of Medicine

DECEMBER 16 DEADLINE
Charles E. Schmidt College of Medicine at Florida Atlantic University
Florida International University Herbert Wertheim College of Medicine
Howard University College of Medicine (Regular M.D.)
Indiana University School of Medicine
Meharry Medical College School of Medicine
New York Medical College
Ponce School of Medicine and Health Sciences
San Juan Bautista School of Medicine
Temple University School of Medicine
The Commonwealth Medical College
Tulane University School of Medicine (Regular M.D.)
Universidad Central Del Caribe School of Medicine
Wayne State University School of Medicine (Regular M.D.)

DECEMBER 31 DEADLINE
University of Illinois College of Medicine (M.D.-Ph.D.)

*Deadline dates change frequently. Check the AAMC website often to avoid missing an important date.

Once you have determined what program to pursue, it is time to answer two questions:

1. To how many schools should I apply?

2. To which schools should I apply?

The number of schools depends on the strength of your application. I generally suggest 15-20 for strong applicants, 20-30 for average applicants, and >30 for applicants with low grades/MCAT scores or holes in the application. For re-applicants, I generally recommend 40 schools in addition to osteopathic (DO) and foreign schools.

Where to apply depends on what you are looking for in a medical education. Every medical school in the United States will give you a good education. The decision often comes down to location, people, curriculum, financial aid, residency success, extracurriculars, and overall gut feeling. Though I can't tell you exactly where to apply, here are some suggestions:

- Apply to your state school(s). These schools often offer the best chance of admissions and most affordable way to obtain a medical education.
- Apply to your alma mater if it has a medical school.
- Focus on your state school(s), mid-tier private schools, and a few reach schools unless you are an exceptional candidate.
- Avoid out-of-state public schools unless you have a stellar application. They are often harder to get into than top-tier private schools.
- Apply only to schools you will attend if accepted.
- Think about where you want to live for four+ years.
- Analyze your own learning style. Do you learn better in lecture classes or small groups? Medical schools now vary dramatically in their educational styles with some schools relying heavily on student-driven learning while others take a more traditional lecture-based approach.
- Talk to everyone you know in the medical profession. Where did Aunt Betty go to school and why? What about your family doctor?
- Ask your college's pre-med advisor if he keeps any records of medical schools attended by alumni. See if you can contact alumni who are current students at schools you are interested in attending.
- Visit a bookstore and browse books that compare individual medical schools.
- Review blogs or ask questions of current medical students on interactive sites such as the Student Doctor Network (http://www.studentdoctor.

net/). Be careful not to get sucked into the anxious, competitive pre-med culture that permeates many of these chat-room style sites.

- Many pre-meds like to create their school list by making a spreadsheet comparing their academic stats with the average GPA and MCAT scores of different schools found in the MSAR. Though this is not a bad way to start evaluating where to apply, remember the GPAs and MCATs listed are averages and medical schools take into account much more than grades when evaluating an applicant. Don't throw a school off your list simply because your academic stats are a tad lower than average. And don't assume a medical school will be a "safety" because you blow their mean GPA and MCAT scores out of the water. There is no such thing as a safety school in medical school admissions.

FOREIGN MEDICAL SCHOOLS

In general, it is easier to transfer an American medical license to a foreign country as opposed to going to a foreign medical school and trying to come back to the US. That being said, some schools (*e.g.*, St. George's University, Ross University) have a relationship with US universities making it easier to return after medical school and obtain a US residency. New partnerships between foreign medical schools and US universities are popping up every year. If you are interested in a foreign medical school, a quick Internet search will reveal a surprising number of options.

If you want to practice medicine in the US, it is best to go to school in the US. However, the only true requirements to work as a doctor here are to train (*i.e.*, do residency) in the US and pass the board exams for your specialty. Thus, you may go to school anywhere you want, take the USMLE exams, and apply to residency as a foreign grad. You will likely not be doing dermatology at Harvard, but you can often get a residency spot in less competitive fields and universities. For more information on foreign schools, please see Appendix VIII.

VIII. Personal Statement

We'll spend the rest of May and some of June tackling this one.

IX. Standardized Tests

An easy, breezy section. All MCAT scores after 2003 will be released to AMCAS automatically. You may add other scores, such as GRE.

MAY WEEK 2
AMCAS: Work/Activities (Section V)

This week is dedicated to completing section V of the AMCAS application known as the work/activities section. Think of the work/activities as an annotated resume highlighting your breadth of accomplishments and introducing the admissions committee to your application story.

In 2011, AMCAS modified the work/activities section requirements. In previous years, AMCAS allowed 15 activities with descriptions totaling 1325 characters each. Now, you still have 15 activity spaces but only 700 characters for each description. In addition, AMCAS requires you to select three "most meaningful" activities out of those listed with additional 1325 characters of explanation allowed. Remember hard returns (enter) count as two characters.

AMCAS categorizes entries as follows:

- Artistic Endeavors
- Community Service/Volunteer – Medical/Clinical
- Community Service/Volunteer – Not Medical/Clinical
- Conferences Attended
- Extracurricular Activities
- Hobbies
- Honors/Awards/Recognitions
- Intercollegiate Athletics
- Leadership – Not Listed Elsewhere
- Military Service
- Other
- Paid Employment – Medical/Clinical
- Paid Employment – Not Medical/Clinical
- Physician Shadowing/Clinical Observation
- Presentations/Posters
- Publications

- Research/Lab
- Teaching/Tutoring/Teaching Assistant

These categories change slightly from year to year, but always focus on allowing applicants to show their well-roundedness.

AMCAS requires you include experience type, experience name, experience dates, total hours, organization name/country/city, and the name/title/phone number/e-mail of a contact that can vouch you participated in the activity. This contact may be a professor, coach, community service advisor, principal investigator, etc. It should not be a member of your family. If the activity relates to a student-organized group with no advisor, you may list a contact in your university's student affairs office to verify participation. If absolutely no contact is known, you can enter a peer or yourself. Use this option as a last resort.

AMCAS frequently changes how it asks for the number of hours you have participated in an activity. It used to request hours/week. Now AMCAS wants total hours, but maxes out the total hours number at 999. Thus, if you participated in an activity for more than 999 hours, you have to enter multiple dates each with 999 hours to add up to your total. Yes, this is confusing. Check out the AMCAS examples below and in Appendix II to see how to enter hours. Hopefully, AMCAS will change this maximum hour limit in the near future to make filling out the application more straightforward.

When filling out the work/activities section, only include significant experiences and avoid repeats. For example, if you shadowed multiple physicians for one day each, create one "shadowing" entry and list the details of each shadowing experience. You can also put all honors/awards/recognitions and publications under their own single entries. Aim to compose an easy-to-read AMCAS work/activities section in the same way you would create a resume. Medical school admissions committee members often breeze through this section quickly. Do note AMCAS automatically lists work/activities entries in chronological order, which may not be rearranged by you. The admissions committees can sort the work/activities section in any order they choose.

There is no need to fill all 15 entries. I rarely allow clients 15 work/activities because, frankly, few pre-meds have 15 exceptional experiences. Medical school admissions committees prefer to see nine stellar work/activities entries rather than 15 mediocre ones. In general, admission committees place more weight on activities showing dedication over a period of time and leadership. They look down on repeats. Don't fill the space just to fill the space.

The change to 700 characters of description plus an additional 1325 characters for most meaningful activities makes the AMCAS work/activities section easier because your experience descriptions may be more concise and resume-like. However, the "most meaningful" activities can be tricky. I suggest picking three accomplishments that emphasize your well-roundedness. For example, choose one research, one community service, and one clinical experience, as opposed to highlighting three research activities. I do suggest writing the "most meaningful" descriptions in proper English in paragraph form. You can use more stunted, resume-like wording in the 700-character experience descriptions. Avoid the "I did this" and then "I learned this" format advocated on some websites. Show what you did and learned instead of telling the committee about it. You want to be direct and nuanced at the same time.

Here are two fictional examples of the AMCAS work/activities section. Which do you find more impressive?

AMCAS Work/Activities Example 1

Experience Type: Paid Employment – Not Medical/Clinical
Most Meaningful Experience: Yes
Experience Name: Eastern African Relief Team Leader
Dates: 09/2009 – 08/2010
Total Hours: 520
Dates: 09/2010 – 08/2011
Total Hours: 750
Dates: 09/2011 – 08/2012
Total Hours: 999
Dates: 09/2012 – present
Total Hours: 999
Contact Name & Title: Dr. David Dogood, Chairman, Relief Services
Contact E-mail: dogood@google.com
Contact Phone: 555-444-5359
Organization Name: Care For All
City/State/Country: Washington, DC, USA
Experience Description: During my first year of college, I joined the Care for All Relief Services Division as an office assistant in attempt to gain a sense

of methods used by large organizations handling overhead and organizational challenges of international relief missions. The work so engaged me that I have stayed with the organization throughout my college career and have been promoted from office assistant to African Relief Team assistant to Eastern African Relief Team leader. Now, as the full-time Eastern African Relief Team Leader, I coordinate the fund-raising, volunteer, and distribution efforts of relief missions directed to the Eastern African continent.

Most Meaningful Experience Remarks: Working at Care for All has confirmed my desire to specialize in international healthcare delivery with a particular focus on Africa. Adding medical knowledge and clinical skills to my growing understanding of how to best help those in the developing world, I look forward to making a direct impact on the poorest of the poor. In addition, moving up in the company has improved my understanding of organizational structure and leadership skills. The work has been challenging and even frustrating at times, such as when bureaucracy impedes progress, but these trials have only left me more motivated to create change in a positive way for those most in need.

Experience Type: Intercollegiate Athletics
Most Meaningful Experience: Yes
Experience Name: Varsity Swimming
Dates: 09/2009 – 05/2010
Total Hours: 999
Dates: 09/2010 – 05/2011
Total Hours: 999
Dates: 09/2011 – 05/2012
Total Hours: 999
Dates: 09/2012 – 05/2013
Total Hours: 999
Contact Name & Title: Coach Carly Carlile, Head Women's Swimming Coach
Contact E-mail: swim@google.com
Contact Phone: 555-554-5858
Organization Name: Maryland College Swimming (Captain)
City/State/Country: Potomac, Maryland, USA
Experience Description: Four-year member of three-time Eastern Athletic Conference Championship Team. Elected captain for 2012-2013 season. All-American in 200-meter individual medley 2011, 2012, 2013.

Most Meaningful Experience Remarks: As a four-year member of Maryland College's Varsity Swim Team, I learned the power of time management, perseverance, and leadership. I spent an average of 40-60 hours per week swimming, weight lifting, and watching film and quickly learned the discipline required to maintain my athletic, academic, research, and community service commitments. Instead of trying to do everything, I learned to give my full attention and longitudinal commitment to fewer meaningful tasks. After an injury to my rotator cuff junior year, I battled through the pain and disappointment to win the National Championship in the 200-meter individual medley. Honored to be named captain my senior year, I enjoyed leading our team to another stellar year, winning the conference title and placing in the top ten at nationals.

Experience Type: Community Service/Volunteer – Medical/Clinical
Most Meaningful Experience: No
Experience Name: Emergency Department Volunteer
Dates: 09/2009 – 05/2013
Total Hours: 999
Contact Name & Title: Mrs. Val Vinson, Volunteer Coordinator
Contact E-mail: valv@google.com
Contact Phone: 555-121-3245
Organization Name: City Hospital
City/State/Country: Washington, DC, USA
Experience Description: Emergency department volunteer for four years. Elected volunteer supervisor during senior year. Tasks included assisting physicians with basic procedures, performing CPR during codes, providing food/blankets to patients and families, and patient transport.

Experience Type: Research/Lab
Most Meaningful Experience: Yes
Experience Name: Research Assistant
Dates: 10/2009 – 05/2011
Total Hours: 999
Dates: 09/2011 – 05/2013
Total Hours: 999
Contact Name & Title: Dr. Earnest Everest, Principal Investigator

Contact E-mail: earnest@google.com
Contact Phone: 555-333-5350
Organization Name: Incite Research Lab
City/State/Country: Potomac, Maryland, USA
Experience Description: Joined the Incite Research Lab as a research assistant in 2009 where I performed PCR analysis and electrophoresis on DNA from HIV patients resistant to Combivir antiretroviral medication. With the assistance of Dr. Everest, designed and obtained NIH funding for my own project investigating the medication resistance patterns of HIV patients undergoing direct observational therapy versus self-directed therapy in Somalia. The findings were recently published in Analysis (8(21):1928-1938, March 2013).
Most Meaningful Experience Remarks: Working in Dr. Everest's lab four all four years of college allowed me to grow from an initially untrained research assistant into a published independent researcher. I started assisting the lab's post-docs and learning the technical skills required to perform biochemical research. After mastering the technical skills, I dove into the problem-solving aspect of research, offering my ideas at weekly lab meetings and journal clubs. By my second year in the lab, I devised my own project and obtained NIH funding. I completed the project over the next two years and was published in Analysis in 2013. I hope to merge the research skills learned in the lab with my knowledge of international health delivery to devise models to best assess how to provide care for Africa's underserved populations.

Experience Type: Conferences Attended
Most Meaningful Experience: No
Experience Name: National and International Conferences
Dates: 10/2010 – 03/2013
Total Hours: 200
Contact Name & Title: Dr. Earnest Everest, Principal Investigator
Contact E-mail: earnest@google.com
Contact Phone: 555-333-5350
Organization Name: Incite Research Lab
City/State/Country: Potomac, Maryland, USA
Experience Description: Through my work with the Incite Research Lab, I attended the following national and international conferences focused on HIV science:

International Association of HIV Researchers, October 2010, Cape Town, South Africa

HIV Science Exposition, May 2011, Melbourne, Australia

HIV Researchers for a Cure, September 2011, Delhi, India

International Association of HIV Researchers, US Division Meeting, May 2012, New York, New York

National Association of HIV Researchers, March 2013, San Francisco, California

AMCAS Work/Activities Example 2

Experience Type: Extracurricular Activities
Most Meaningful Experience: No
Experience Name: Club Member
Dates: 09/2010 – 5/2011
Total Hours: 40
Contact Name & Title: Mr. Stu Simpson, Faculty Supervisor
Contact E-mail: stu@google.com
Contact Phone: 555-823-5858
Organization Name: Maryland College Pre-Medical Society
City/State/Country: Potomac, Maryland, USA
Experience Description: Member of Maryland College Pre-Medical Society

Experience Type: Artistic Endeavors
Most Meaningful Experience: No
Experience Name: Singer
Dates: 09/2010 – 12/2010
Total Hours: 24
Contact Name & Title: Ms. August Aria, Musical Director
Contact E-mail: sing@google.com
Contact Phone: 555-222-2222
Organization Name: A Cappella Are US
City/State/Country: Potomac, Maryland, USA
Experience Description: Member of a cappella group specializing in classic jazz and do-op.

Experience Type: Honors/Awards/Recognitions
Most Meaningful Experience: No
Experience Name: Dean's List
Dates: 09/2010 – 05/2011
Total Hours: 0
Contact Name & Title: Mrs. Sue Sullivan, Registrar
Contact E-mail: sue@google.com
Contact Phone: 555-757-5858
Organization Name: Maryland College
City/State/Country: Potomac, Maryland, USA
Experience Description: Made Dean's List first year of college.

Experience Type: Paid Employment – Not Medical/Clinical
Most Meaningful Experience: No
Experience Name: Retail Employee
Dates: 01/2011 – 05/2011
Total Hours: 100
Contact Name & Title: Mr. Yan Yogi, Store Manager
Contact E-mail: yogi@google.com
Contact Phone: 555-234-5435
Organization Name: Fashion Diva
City/State/Country: Potomac, Maryland, USA
Experience Description: Worked part-time in Fashion Diva Apparel Store to help meet college expenses.

Experience Type: Community Service/Volunteer – Not Medical/Clinical
Most Meaningful Experience: No
Experience Name: Volunteer
Dates: 12/2011 – 12/2011
Total Hours: 3
Contact Name & Title: Mrs. Mary Munsey, Director
Contact E-mail: mary@google.com
Contact Phone: 555-554-5346
Organization Name: Potomac Soup Kitchen
City/State/Country: Potomac, Maryland, USA

Experience Description: Served Christmas dinner to the homeless at Potomac Soup Kitchen.

Experience Type: Research/Lab
Most Meaningful Experience: Yes
Experience Name: Research Assistant
Dates: 01/2012– 05/2012
Total Hours: 100
Contact Name & Title: Dr. Cal Cerebro, Principal Investigator
Contact E-mail: cerebro@google.com
Contact Phone: 555-234-7544
Organization Name: Neuroscience Laboratories of Maryland
City/State/Country: Potomac, Maryland, USA
Experience Description: Performed electrophoresis studies on mouse DNA for project investigating the effect of sleeplessness on telomere shortening.
Most Meaningful Experience Remarks: I joined Dr. Cerebro's lab to gain technical research skills and hone my problem-solving ability. For a semester, I assisted the lab's post-docs by performing electrophoresis studies on mouse DNA. The work took patience and attention to detail. I particularly enjoyed learning about the day-to-day life of a researcher and attending monthly lab meetings. I left the lab when the school year ended.

Experience Type: Teaching/Tutoring/Teaching Assistant
Most Meaningful Experience: Yes
Experience Name: Tutor
Dates: 09/2012 – 05/2013
Total Hours: 78
Contact Name & Title: Mrs. Hattie Hanson, Supervisor
Contact E-mail: hattie@google.com
Contact Phone: 555-442-5858
Organization Name: Helping Hands
City/State/Country: Potomac, Maryland, USA
Experience Description: Tutored autistic pre-schoolers at the Helping Hands School. Focused on reading comprehension skills.
Most Meaningful Experience Remarks: After reading reports about the

increased incidence of autism in recent years, I decided to tutor autistic children in an attempt to better understand the spectrum of disease and help a population often left behind by the public school system. Over a school year, I visited Helping Hands School weekly to tutor Billy, age 3, and Haddie, age 5. Initially intimidated by their outbursts and decreased interaction compared to other children their age, I quickly learned to enjoy the challenge of engaging Billy and Haddie in learning exercises. The experience certainly honed my patience and has increased my interest in entering a medical field focused on addressing the needs of disabled children.

Experience Type: Publications
Most Meaningful Experience: No
Experience Name: Author
Dates: 10/2012 – 10/2012
Total Hours: 15
Contact Name & Title: Mr. Bif Bergman, Editor-in-Chief
Contact E-mail: bif@google.com
Contact Phone: 555-329-5858
Organization Name: Maryland College Gazette
City/State/Country: Potomac, Maryland, USA
Experience Description: Wrote article entitled, "Why Everyone Should Be a Physician" published in the opinion section of college's weekly newspaper.

Experience Type: Conferences Attended
Most Meaningful Experience: No
Experience Name: Conference Attendee
Dates: 06/2013 – 06/2013
Total Hours: 40
Contact Name & Title: Ms. Bonnie Bumble, Director
Contact E-mail: bonnie@google.com
Contact Phone: 555-234-5234
Organization Name: Maryland College Pre-Medical Conference
City/State/Country: Potomac, Maryland, USA
Experience Description: Attended summer conference sponsored by the Maryland College Pre-Medical Society focusing on careers available in the medical profession.

Experience Type: Community Service/Volunteer – Medical/Clinical
Most Meaningful Experience: Yes
Experience Name: Hospital Volunteer
Dates: 06/2013 – 09/2013
Total Hours: 36
Contact Name & Title: Dr. Frank Feters, Director
Contact E-mail: frank@google.com
Contact Phone: 555-754-6976
Organization Name: Suburban Clinic
City/State/Country: Potomac, Maryland, USA
Experience Description: I volunteered one afternoon per week at the Suburban Clinic, a free walk-in clinic serving the homeless population of Potomac. Took patient histories and vital signs and then reported each patient's information to Dr. Feters.
Most Meaningful Experience Remarks: Volunteering at the Suburban Clinic solidified my desire to become a physician. Every week, I joined Dr. Feters in this free clinic serving a homeless population often suffering from mental illness, substance abuse, and chronic disease. I enjoyed learning from Dr. Feters how to engage and best help this at-risk population and developing long-term relationships with return patients. Dr. Feters allowed me to be an integral part of the care team and taught me how to take histories and vital signs. I hope to continue serving such at-risks populations as a medical student and physician.

Experience Type: Physcian Shadowing/Clinical Observation
Most Meaningful Experience: No
Experience Name: Physician Shadowing
Dates: 01/2014 – 01/2014
Total Hours: 40
Contact Name & Title: Dr. Dean Dannenburg, Physician
Contact E-mail: dean@google.com
Contact Phone: 555-404-5858
Organization Name: Dannenburg Dermatology Associates
City/State/Country: Rockville, Maryland, USA
Experience Description: Shadowed Dr. Dannenburg in his office. Observed both initial and follow-up visits. Also saw multiple procedures including mole removal and Botox application.

Get my drift? Although the second example fills in the space with double the number of activities, I am sure you will agree the first example is more impressive. Admissions committees prefer quality to quantity. Avoid using "one-offs," or experiences you only had one time, to pad the application. Appendix II contains examples of AMCAS and TMDSAS work/activities from successful applicants. Read these examples for inspiration and direction before you start your own work/activities.

AMCAS WORK/ACTIVITIES TIPS

- You are allowed a maximum of 15 experiences with 700 characters to describe each experience.
- Three "most meaningful" experiences must be selected with an additional 1325 characters of explanation allowed.
- Hard returns (enter) count as two characters.
- Medical school admissions committees place more weight on activities that show dedication over a period of time and leadership.
- The admissions committees look down on repeats.
- Don't fill the space just to fill the space. Ten stellar activities are better than 15 less-than-impressive activities.
- AMCAS automatically lists the activities by date.

MAY WEEK 3
AMCAS: Personal Statement Brainstorm (Section VIII)

Section VIII of the AMCAS application is arguably the most important. In the personal statement you are asked to consider the following questions:

- Why have you selected the field of medicine?
- What motivates you to learn more about the field of medicine?
- What information do you want medical schools to know about you that has not been disclosed in another section of the application?

The application also states you:

"May wish to include information such as: Special hardships, challenges, or obstacles that may have influenced your educational pursuits. Commentary on significant fluctuations in your academic record, which are not explained elsewhere in the application."

In other words, you have 5300 characters to say why you want to be a doctor and why an admissions committee should accept you into its medical school class. And you must do this in an interesting, creative, and honest way. This is not an easy task.

Although daunting, the personal statement is also an exciting opportunity. This is one of the few parts of the application you can currently control. At this point, you can't control past grades or MCAT scores, what a recommender has written, or your previous activities. But you can control every word of the personal statement. In about one page, you will explain why you want to be a physician and why you will be an exceptional addition to the medical profession. The personal statement may also serve to highlight interesting talents that may not be readily apparent in other parts of the application.

MD/PhD candidates, please be aware that you have two additional essays to write. The first essay will discuss your reasons for wishing to pursue an MD/PhD (3,000 characters). The second asks for details on your research experience (10,000 characters).

The biggest mistake I have seen medical school applicants make is spending too little time on the personal statement. Creating a memorable personal statement cannot be completed in one sitting. You should set aside at least two weeks and preferably a month to write the statement. Expect to go through at least ten drafts. Be sure to allow time for a pre-med advisor, writing teacher, and/or admissions consultant to give comments on the essay.

Volumes and volumes have been written on the art of crafting an excellent personal statement. I will not attempt to recreate such works here. However, I will provide you with the tips I give my clients. Before you start writing, I suggest performing three brainstorming exercises:

I. Start by making a list of the reasons you want to attend medical school. Likely, some of your top reasons will include, "I like science" and "I like helping people." Hopefully, everyone going to medical school has these two motivations. The trick is holding onto these two reasons while delving deeper into why they are true. When writing your list, ask what life experiences support the reasons you are giving. After writing the list, determine which reason and experience pairs make the strongest argument for why you want to be a physician. This will serve as the basis of your essay. Remember, the list doesn't have to be fancy or use perfect grammar. You are just sketching out some ideas before starting to write. Here's an example of a brainstorm list:

I want to be a physician because:

A. I want to use a team approach to solve problems
Experience:
  - Captain of basketball team that won three league championships
  - Showed how efforts of many can achieve great goals

B. I want to use cutting-edge technology to improve lives
Experience:
  - Research assistant with Dr. Buck at Maryland State University
  - Saw value of PET scanning as it guided diagnosis and treatment of various cancers

C. I want to work in international health and public policy
Experience:
  - Realized a great passion for international health after a mission trip with church to San Juan Sacatapequez, Guatemala
  - Built clinic and trained local nurses in basic sanitary measures
  - Volunteered to raise money for Healthcare for All
  - Joined university's public policy club

D. I want to combine my interest in business and medicine to create more cost-effective and efficient hospitals that provide the best possible care
Experience:
  - Worked as a healthcare consultant at an international consulting firm for the past two years
  - Though enjoyed analyzing focal health care problems of hospital and pharmaceutical companies, I realized the only way to truly understand the challenges of today's health care system is to be an intimate part of it

- As practicing physician, will be better able to pinpoint problems and derive plausible solutions

E. I want to do research that translates from bench to bedside

Experience:

- Worked for two years with Dr. Han creating new HIV drugs that target reverse transcriptase
- Published in *Analytics* last month
- Volunteer in HIV clinic weekly to see how HIV patients respond to drugs currently available

Get the point? Every reason for going to medical school has to be backed up with personal experience. The admissions officer who reads the essay (along with hundreds of other essays) may not remember you want to be a global health physician. But he may remember that you pursued this interest by organizing an aid trip to Indonesia after the tsunami.

II. Think of the personal statement in terms of the characteristics it will show you possess. A list of traits and skills we all look for in good doctors includes:

Psychological maturity

Character and integrity

Self-discipline

Judgment

Compassion and empathy

Communication skills

Concern for helping others

Intellectual curiosity and enthusiasm

Analytical and problem-solving ability

Motivation and persistence

Reliability and dependability

Resilience and adaptability

Accountability

Leadership skills

Teamwork skills

Experience with and knowledge of medicine

When deciding what experiences to include in the essay, think about the characteristics they support.

III. Come up with a great "hook"—an opening that will keep your reader engaged and make her want to read past the first paragraph. A compelling hook frequently includes a good anecdote. Be creative, but be very careful with humor or over-the-top stories. The hook then leads to your thesis statement.

Here are some examples of great hooks:

> Could you invent a vocal part that sounds like a cross between Pink Floyd and K.D. Lang? We need a spectacular finish for the song." I breathed deeply and stepped to the microphone, not yet knowing what to sing. I had first heard this song only an hour before and could feel the songwriter and the album producer listening from outside the recording booth. This is just another type of problem to solve, I reminded myself; listen to how the parts fit together and the answer will come. I began to sing, drawing on my decades of musical experience, and wove my voice among the parts to create a new complete whole.

> Shifting in his chair, chattering about the warm weather, and avoiding eye contact, the man across from me exuded anxiety. I did not know why Ben had come to a HIV counselor, but I realized direct questioning would not help me find out. I started by addressing the present moment and that he seemed anxious. As we chatted, Ben turned toward me, slowed his speech, and looked me in the eye revealing that he may have exposed his partner to HIV. After we made a connection and discussed the options, Ben left the counseling session with a cautious resolve to talk frankly with his partner. This counseling interaction exemplifies qualities I will bring to the practice of medicine: the ability to build trust, to respond to people on their own terms, and to see patients as situated in biological, psychological, and cultural contexts.

Personal statement examples written by previous MDadmit clients and colleagues are included in Appendix I. Each essay highlights a different way of creating a unique and memorable personal statement.

AMCAS PERSONAL STATEMENT BIGGEST MISTAKES

Spending too little time on statement

Simply repeating AMCAS work/activities

Weak thesis

Poor transition sentences

Overly informal tone

Inappropriate use of humor

Over-reliance on quotes

Poor grammar or typos

MAY WEEK 4
AMCAS: Personal Statement Drafts 1-3

Once you have completed the three brainstorming tasks, it is time to write your first draft. Don't spend too much time on this—just write. Don't focus on grammar yet. Put the essay away for a day, and then come back with a critical eye to content and write a second draft. Does this one page of words summarize why you want to be a physician? Put the essay away for another day and then write your third draft, focusing on both content and grammar.

After the third draft, it is time to send out the essay for an expert opinion—choose two or three people with experience in writing personal statements and gather their thoughts on three things: content, grammar, and flow (how easily the essay reads). Afraid you don't know anyone who can edit the essay for you? Don't be—they surround you. Try your parents, spouse, friend who majored in English, cousin in medical school, career counselor, university writing service, writing instructor, family physician, coach, admissions consultant, *etc*. If you think hard enough, I know you can find two or three people willing to give comments on your essay. Don't be afraid to ask. Most people will think of it as an honor. One word of caution—do not send the essay to too many people for opinions. Readers will undoubtedly disagree, and it can be very frustrating trying to please everyone. The only two people you have to please are yourself and the admissions officer.

CHECKLIST

❏ Complete AMCAS sections I-IV, VI, VII, and IX

❏ Complete AMCAS work/activities (section V)

❏ Brainstorm personal statement (section VIII)

❏ Complete first three drafts of personal statement

NOTES

June Year 1
Finish and Submit AMCAS

"What is written without effort is in general read without pleasure."
-SAMUEL JOHNSON

Ideally, you want to submit your final AMCAS application in June. It does not need to be the very first day AMCAS opens, which ranges from June 1 to June 10 depending on the year. AMCAS usually does not begin transmitting information to medical schools until the end of June. Submit the best application possible around mid-June to allow two to six weeks for processing and still have one of the first applications transmitted to the medical schools. Submitting early gives you a dramatic advantage in rolling admissions schools. Though early submission is less important for non-rolling admission schools, getting your application in so that you can receive secondary applications and then interviews early also tends to help increase your chance of admission. Submitting the AMCAS in June also allows time to troubleshoot if something goes wrong such as a technical error or a missing recommendation. Early submission is equally important for TMDSAS and AACOMAS applications.

JUNE WEEK 1
AMCAS: Personal Statement Drafts 4-6

You now have written three personal statement drafts and received comments from at least two readers. Be sure to say thank you to those who read the essay and then put on your thick skin. There will surely be negative comments (that's the whole point of asking someone to edit the essay). The remarks will certainly not all be in agreement. This is your essay. Own it. Take all the observations constructively and choose the ones you believe will best improve the essay.

Turn out a fourth draft of the personal statement incorporating your editors' comments. Put the essay away for a day and then return for the fifth draft. Put it away again and then edit only for grammar, creating the sixth draft. Send this sixth draft back to your editors for last thoughts on content and flow. Once you have completed the sixth draft, return to the AMCAS work/activities section again and edit for grammar and typos.

JUNE WEEK 2
AMCAS: Personal Statement Drafts 7-8

Respond to the comments on content and flow in seventh and eighth drafts, taking a day off in between to regain perspective. When the eighth draft is complete, send it to a copy editor—either a professional or a person you know who possesses meticulous attention to detail and strong knowledge of grammar. The goal is to edit for typos and grammar as opposed to content.

JUNE WEEK 3
AMCAS: Personal Statement Drafts 9-10 and Submission

Sick of this personal statement yet? You are close to finishing, so hang in there. When the copy edits return, complete a ninth draft by performing a final edit for content, grammar, and flow. Put the essay away for a day. Then, before you submit the AMCAS, do a final copy edit of the essay. This will be your tenth draft. Copy edit the entire AMCAS application and then submit it electronically. Congrats! You have officially applied to medical school and are on your way to earning a MD.

JUNE WEEK 4
AMCAS: Recommendations Check

Now that the AMCAS is submitted (breathe a huge and well-deserved sigh of relief), contact all of your recommenders/pre-med committee/recommendation service (*e.g.,* AMCAS, Interfolio, VirtualEvals) to ensure the letters of evaluation have been sent out and received. Many schools will not process your AMCAS application until all recommendations are received.

CHECKLIST

❑ Complete personal statement

❑ Copy edit entire AMCAS application

❑ Submit AMCAS application

❑ Check on recommendations

NOTES

July Year 1

Secondary Applications

*"Either write something worth reading
or do something worth writing."*
-BEN FRANKLIN

S econdary applications, or secondaries, are sent individually from each medical school once the AMCAS application has been received. Many schools use the AMCAS as an initial screening, and then send secondaries to obtain more information from applicants in order to determine who receives an interview. Some will only send a secondary to applicants who meet certain requirements (often based on GPA and MCAT scores). Other schools automatically generate a secondary upon receipt of your AMCAS application. This is quickly becoming the norm, especially for private schools. Once the AMCAS is certified, secondaries will stagger into your inbox over the next few months.

Secondaries vary greatly in substance. Some require nothing more than your name and a check (average secondary charge is $75). Others entail up to 10 essays and are very time consuming. The due date varies by school. It is best to turn in a secondary as soon as possible after receiving it in order to move the admissions process along. Be aware that some schools put very tight deadlines on secondaries, as short as one week from the time the application is e-mailed.

Though schools change their secondary essay prompts from year to year, most of the questions fall into 12 broad categories that I will list in the next three months' chapters. Instead of writing a new answer to each question for every school, I suggest you compose answers to each of these 12 questions and morph them as needed to a particular application. This will save you both time and energy. It also gives you a chance to write exceptional essays that may be used multiple times with minor tweaking. Most of the secondary essays range from 250-500 words. I suggest writing an answer to each question listed below in 250-500 words, and then editing as needed to fit each particular application's word requirement. The sample questions provided have been modified from real secondary applications. Get that literary mind going because you may have hundreds of secondary essays to write in the next few months. Appendix III provides examples of secondary question answers to inspire your personal brainstorm on how to approach the most common topics.

MOST COMMON SECONDARY ESSAY TOPICS

Diversity
How will you add a unique dimension to our medical school community?

Personal Challenge/Ethical Dilemma
Describe a challenge you have overcome and what you learned from the experience.

After-College Activities
If you have already graduated, briefly summarize your activities since graduation.

Specific School Interest
Indicate the reasons for your specific interest in Man's Greatest Medical School.

Most Important Activity
From among the activities and experiences listed in your AMCAS application, please select one activity that has most impacted your decision to enter medicine.

Research
What self-education, research, or independent academic work have you performed and what have you accomplished in this work?

Long-Term Goals
Are there any areas of medicine that are of particular interest to you?

Qualities/Characteristics
Describe the distinguishable characteristics you possess. How will these characteristics enhance your success as a medical student and future physician?

Most Important Relationship
Who is the most influential person in your life and why?

Autobiographical/Personal Insight
Write another essay that provides us with some insight into you as a person.

Academic Awards
Please list collegiate honors, awards, and memberships in honorary societies.

Other Information
Is there any other information you would like to share with the admissions committee?

JULY WEEK 1
Secondaries: Diversity

Diversity is one of the most popular secondary essay topics. In answering the following questions, you want to show how you will make a unique contribution to the medical school class.

Here are some examples from secondary applications:

1. We are committed to building a diverse community. What will you as an individual bring to our medical school community?
2. How will you add a unique dimension to our medical school community? What is your greatest strength? What is your greatest weakness?
3. Please describe a situation where you were not in the majority.

When the word "diversity" is used, many think of racial diversity. But this is a very limited view. Do not be concerned if you are not from a minority background—you too can add to the diversity of the class. Perhaps you speak Croatian or are proficient in American Sign Language. That would certainly add diversity to a medical school class. Or maybe, you are a non-traditional applicant who has worked in Silicon Valley for the past five years managing scores of employees. Other possibilities include athletic achievements, musical/art/dance talent, and international experience. Everyone can add diversity to a class. Think outside the box about what sets you apart from other candidates and how this could make a medical school class more interesting.

JULY WEEK 2
Secondaries: Personal Challenge/Ethical Dilemma

Medicine is a challenging profession. Illness and death are a part of daily life. Hours are long. The system is frustrating. (Sounds great, doesn't it?) Admission committees want to know how well you meet challenges and handle ethical dilemmas. You may be asked to:

1. Describe a challenge you have overcome and what you learned from the experience.
2. Describe a personal experience that resulted in a substantial ethical dilemma. Please do not address academic cheating. We will not accept that you have never faced a challenge.
3. Describe a situation in which you were really stressed and relay how you dealt with it.
4. Describe your most humbling experience.

As mentioned in the second topic, everyone has overcome a challenge. It is not acceptable to state that your life has been peachy keen and nothing has ever gone wrong. In others words, you can't leave this one blank. You may provide an answer from any area of your life—personal, professional, extracurricular, *etc.* Be careful not to be too sappy in your answer. You don't have to be the hero. The key is showing how you came to a decision during a challenging situation and what you learned from it.

JULY WEEK 3
Secondaries: After-College Activities

Now that taking time off before medical school is completely accepted (and often encouraged), many secondaries ask about after-college activities:

1. Please indicate your activities for the xxxx-yyyy year.
2. If you have already graduated, briefly summarize your activities since graduation.
3. What have you done since college?

Obviously, if you are still in college when applying to medical school, you will leave this type of question blank unless otherwise specified. If you have just graduated, feel free to discuss your summer activities and upcoming plans before matriculation into medical school. And if you have taken time off, use this section to flesh out what you have done more fully than was allowed on the AMCAS work/activities list.

JULY WEEK 4
Secondaries: Specific School Interest

Many schools like to know that you want them. The Columbia dean of admissions mentioned during the interview that sending a letter of intent would increase my chance of admission. Most schools won't be so honest, but the sentiment is similar across institutions—they want to be wanted. Why? Many schools publish admissions statistics including the percentage of admissions offers accepted. A school looks more desirable when the vast majority of offers are accepted. Thus, schools often try to determine not only the best applicants, but also the best applicants that will say yes to their offer. This psychology is the basis for very common secondary questions:

1. Indicate the reasons for your specific interest in Man's Greatest Medical School.
2. Why have you chosen to apply to Maryland State School of Medicine, and how do you think your education here will prepare you to become a physician?

Admissions committees are looking for a detailed answer. They want to know you researched their school by visiting the website, talking with current students and graduates, and/or reading published marketing material. Since humans think best in groups of three, I suggest you develop three distinct reasons for each school. Here are some fictional examples that can be expanded into paragraph form to create a strong answer:

- Unique opportunity to continue behavioral science research in Dr. John Lee's Integrated Behavioral Science Laboratory.
- Chance to obtain early clinical exposure by working at HEAL, the student-run free clinic.
- Exposure to diverse patient population given rotations at Man's Greatest Hospital, General Hospital, and The Clinics.
- Urban setting that will allow for continued participation in Modern Dance Company.
- Problem-based learning curriculum that meshes well with learning style.
- Dedicated time to pursue international opportunities through Global Health for All.

CHECKLIST

❑ Draft answers to each of the most common secondary questions

❑ Complete secondaries upon arrival

NOTES

August Year 1

More Secondary Applications

"Words are, of course, the most powerful drug used by mankind."
-RUDYARD KIPLING

Secondary-mania continues in August. See below for continued discussion of the most common secondary application questions.

Reminder: August 1 is the AMCAS deadline for Early Decision Program students. Aren't you glad you turned in the AMCAS application over a month ago? (If you haven't turned it in yet, get a move on.)

AUGUST WEEK 1
Secondaries: Most Important Activity

Many secondary applications ask you to highlight one particular experience listed on the AMCAS. They often ask specifically about clinical exposure or community service. When thinking about which activity to discuss, remember admissions committees are often more impressed with experiences involving consistent commitment, leadership, or unique circumstances. Examples of most important activity questions include:

1. From among the activities and experiences listed in your AMCAS application, please select one activity that has most impacted your decision to enter medicine.
2. What has been your most important exposure to clinical medicine?

3. What was the single most meaningful volunteer experience you have had?

4. Briefly describe your most rewarding experience or some achievement of which you are particularly proud.

5. Please check up to three activities that are most important to you and describe how they helped you develop skills in leadership and commitment.

When answering this type of question, do not simply repeat information already included on the AMCAS application. Start by briefly summarizing the activity, and then delve into deeper detail about how the experience affected you as a person.

AUGUST WEEK 2
Secondaries: Research

Some questions focus specifically on research or scholarly activities:

1. Although research is not a prerequisite for admission to Man's Greatest Medical School, if you have participated in a scholarly project please describe it here.

2. What self-education, research, or independent academic work have you performed and what have you have accomplished in this work?

Don't panic if you have not published in *Nature* or performed amazing bench research. "Research" is a broad term. In addition to basic science research, medical schools want to hear about your investigations in public health, health policy, and international health. I took the meaning even farther in my application and discussed working as a research assistant for a history professor. The key is to show a proficiency gathering and analyzing data, whether that's data on reverse transcriptase or the first female Nobel Prize winner.

AUGUST WEEK 3
Secondaries: Long-Term Goals

Another favorite secondary question asks about long-term goals (*i.e.*, what you want to be when you grow up). Though you are certainly not expected to have chosen your specialty and fellowship before entering medical school, admissions committees like to know where you are leaning. Do you see yourself working as a general surgeon at a large academic center? Or perhaps you'd like to run a small, rural family medicine clinic. Or maybe you want to be a flight doctor for the Navy. The sky is the limit. But be honest and ready to back up your dream job. Remember, the admissions committee will not follow you to fourth year of medical school to see what specialty you choose. For example, I went to medical school expecting to become an orthopedic surgeon and ended up falling in love with emergency medicine. Answer the question to the best of your ability at this stage of your life.

1. Are there any areas of medicine that are of particular interest to you?
2. In a brief paragraph, please describe how you would want to be remembered at the end of your life.
3. What satisfactions do you expect to receive from your activities as a physician?
4. What is the most likely practice scenario for you in the future? Pick one of the following that best fits your career goals: academic medicine, private practice, health policy, health administration, public health, and global health.

This fourth question can be particularly tricky because many applicants have interests in multiple fields. Pick the area that most intrigues you to adequately answer the question, and then feel free to briefly discuss other interests. Always ensure the question is actually answered in your essay.

AUGUST WEEK 4
Secondaries: Qualities/Characteristics

Medical schools love to ask about qualities you possess that will make you a great physician:

1. Describe the distinguishable characteristics you possess. How will these characteristics enhance your success as a medical student and future physician?

2. In addition to academic achievement, what do you believe are the three most important qualities a physician must have to be successful in medicine and why?
3. Describe the personal characteristics and values (*e.g.,* commitment, integrity, compassion) that make you a suitable candidate for medicine.

When thinking about these questions, review the characteristics and skills list discussed in the personal statement brainstorming section (May Year 1, Week 3):

Psychological maturity
Character and integrity
Self-discipline
Judgment
Compassion and empathy
Communication skills
Concern for helping others
Intellectual curiosity and enthusiasm
Analytical and problem-solving ability
Motivation and persistence
Reliability and dependability
Resilience and adaptability
Accountability
Leadership skills
Teamwork skills
Experience with and knowledge of medicine

This list is certainly not exhaustive but gives you a sense of the kind of qualities and skills medical schools expect you to possess.

Do you notice how many of these questions ask for three characteristics? Humans think best in groups of three. For any secondary answer, it is often useful to break up your answer into three succinct points.

CHECKLIST

❑ Complete secondaries upon arrival

NOTES

September Year 1

Even More Secondary Applications

"All the fun is in how you say a thing."
-ROBERT FROST

By September, you are probably quite fatigued from writing secondaries. Those of you who applied to 30+ schools are likely close to burning out at this point. Keep your focus. Secondaries received now are as important as those received in July. This month discusses four more common secondary essay questions.

SEPTEMBER WEEK 1
Secondaries: Most Important Relationship

In true touchy-feely style, some medical school secondary essays like to ask about the most important relationship in your life. For example:

1. Who is the most influential person in your life and why?
2. What relationship in your life has best prepared you for a career as a physician?

It can be quite hard to answer this question without sounding a bit cheesy. Feel free to think outside the box. The answer does not need to include a family member, even though it is completely appropriate to do so. What about coaches, community service advisors, mentors, or patients? Do not feel the need to write about your mom or family physician. Creativity can work very well with these types of broad questions.

SEPTEMBER WEEK 2
Secondaries: Autobiographical/Personal Insight

I am sorry if one of the following secondary questions lands in your inbox:

1. Give a picture of yourself, your family, and events you consider important to you while identifying the values of greatest importance to you.
2. Write another essay that provides us with some insight into you as a person.

Really? You want my autobiography? Sadly, yes. They really do. The key to answering such an expansive question is to hit the highlights and keep it concise. Word limits are often given; be sure to stay within them. And don't drone on about your family and education history. Offer specific examples and anecdotes to keep the audience interested. For example, you may start with an amusing story from your childhood that foreshadows the kind of adult you are to become. My mother loves to tell the story of my string bracelet business started at age seven. After creating the hand-made merchandise, I walked into a neighborhood sports store and asked the man behind the counter to carry the product. To my mother's shock, the PJs Sport and Surf manager said yes and sold the bracelets for a year. This story from my youth portrays me as intelligent, confident, and creative, three characteristics that look good to admissions committees. I am sure you have similar stories that will launch excellent answers to these very difficult autobiographical/personal insight questions.

SEPTEMBER WEEK 3
Secondaries: Academic Awards

Finally, straightforward secondary essay questions:

1. Please list collegiate honors, awards, and memberships in honorary societies.
2. List any academic honors or awards you have received since entering college.

That's it. Just list the awards. Research grants, community service awards, and extracurricular honors should be included as well.

SEPTEMBER WEEK 4
Secondaries: "Other" Information

Many medical schools will end the secondary application with a question such as:

1. Please share with us something about yourself not addressed elsewhere in your application.
2. Is there any other information you would like to share with the admissions committee?
3. We no longer require a secondary essay, but some applicants feel additional information is required to provide us with a better understanding of who they are as a person and why they will be exceptional physicians. The essay is completely optional. Please do not repeat information found on the AMCAS application.

The "other" information question often causes great stress among candidates. Given that it's usually an optional essay, the big issue is whether or not to answer it. Only answer the question if you have personal information not provided on the AMCAS that will affect your application. Here are a few examples of appropriate topics for this essay:

1. Extenuating circumstances led to a dip in your grades sophomore year and you want to explain.
2. Your band cut its first record after the AMCAS submission.
3. You have a paper accepted for publication that occurred after AMCAS submission.

4. You just received an offer to travel to Africa with a public health project.

Do not fill the space just to fill the space. Only answer the question if you really have something important to say that will positively affect your application.

CHECKLIST

❑ Complete secondaries upon arrival

NOTES

October Year 1

The Interview Trail:
Scheduling and Style Prep

"In matters of style, swim with the current;
in matters of principle, stand like a rock."
-THOMAS JEFFERSON

Though you still may be swamped with secondaries, interview season has begun. Interviews generally span from September to February. Rolling admissions schools tend to interview earlier than others (and let you know of acceptance earlier as well). The next twelve weeks will be dedicated to mastering the art of interviewing. I suggest reading all twelve weeks before your first interview.

All interviews start with a first impression. This means you need to be well dressed and well groomed. Once you are a physician, your patients will want you to look put together. And so do the interviewers. It may seem cliché and shallow, but you need to look good.

OCTOBER WEEK 1
Interviews: Scheduling

Does time of interview really affect chance of acceptance? Yes and no. Yes, if the school does rolling admissions. Rolling admissions schools interview a batch of applicants, and then offer the best candidates admission within weeks. The later you interview, the less spots are available. Interview timing is less critical for regular admissions schools. You will see pages and pages on medical school admissions blogs and forums discussing the best strategic time to interview. Here's the bottom line: interview when you will be well rested and well prepared. This means avoid making your top choice school(s) your first interview or your last or scheduling an interview during hectic exam or work periods..

Be sure to plan for sufficient time off for interview travel, as you want to be fresh and ready to perform your best in each interview. Try to arrive the night before the interview so if you are held up due to transportation problems, you will have adequate time to make secondary plans.

OCTOBER WEEK 2
Interviews: Suit and Shoes

The suit is the wardrobe staple of anyone heading out on the medical school interview trail. Despite popular opinion, it does not have to be black and boring. Yes, doctors tend to be on the more conservative side of the fashion spectrum, but you do not need to give up all style for interviews. I wore a lovely silk deep green suit with black heels that stood out in a good way. The goal should be elegant for the ladies and dapper for the men. Your dad's baby blue tuxedo from the '70s with matching ruffled shirt may be hip, but it's probably a little too stylish. And your sister's four-inch suede miniskirt that looks great with sexy high brown leather boots should probably stay in her closet. I suggest a nice dark (blue, grey, black) tailored suit with cleanly pressed shirt and colorful tie for the gentleman. Ladies, you can pull off either wearing a pantsuit (completely acceptable) or a more traditional suit jacket and skirt combination. Pair the suit with a colorful blouse and simple jewelry, such as stud earrings and a pendant necklace. I know money may be tight, but I do suggest purchasing a nice suit for the interviews. If it is good quality and a classic style, you will use it for the rest of your life. It is acceptable to wear the same suit to every interview. I promise the admissions committees don't compare style notes.

Shoes. You may think it is absurd to dedicate an entire paragraph to interview shoes, but I promise you will thank me later. Shoes are probably the most important part of the interview outfit. These shoes need to be incredibly comfortable, work in various climates, and look classy. I can't tell you how many poor interviewing souls have cursed the shoes they bought for the trail. The Manola Blahnik stilettos will not seem like a good idea after your first three-hour school tour. At some schools, the majority of your interview day will be spent walking. So these shoes need to be comfortable. In addition, if you are interviewing at schools above the Mason Dixon Line in winter, you likely will be walking in snow and ice. Spending the afternoon in the emergency department after cracking your ankle may seem like a good way to get sympathy points, but it will likely just make you look silly. Finally, the shoes need to be easily cleaned or shined so they look new at every interview. An old business interview secret is that shoes are the window to a potential hire's work ethic. Shined, well-kept shoes show a person is detail-oriented and dedicated to an overall polished look. Feel free to scoff, but shoes matter.

OCTOBER WEEK 3
Interviews: Hair and Accessories

The medical school interview season is not the time to experiment with the mohawk you always wanted. Keep hair clean and simple. If you are a man with long hair, you do not need to cut it. Just ensure it is clean and out of your face (same rules apply to women).

As for jewelry, earrings in men are always a point of controversy. If your earring is an important part of who you are, leave it in. But if you consider it just a piece of jewelry, I would take it out. There are certainly old-school doctors out there who don't want to accept an applicant that seems like a "punk." Yes, I know this is incredibly out of date, but your interviewer may come from a time when men wearing earrings was less acceptable. Do you really want to throw away your entire application on a piece of jewelry? If you want to make a statement, make sure you get into medical school first.

Body piercings that show (nose ring, tongue ring, eyebrow ring, *etc.*) fall under the same general guidelines as earrings. Wear it if it is a huge part of who you are. Lose it for a day if it isn't.

OCTOBER WEEK 4
Interviews: First Twelve Inches

To help you pull it all together on your interview day, etiquette experts have a simple rule to ensure you are looking your best. It's the first 12 inches of your head, hands, and feet that matter most:

Head:

Keep the cowlick under control.

Be clean-shaven.

Check teeth for errant vegetable matter and lipstick.

Hands:

Groom nails short and clean.

Chipped nail polish is worse than none at all.

Feet:

Polish your shoes (yes, I actually mean go out and buy real shoe polish and scrub those puppies 'til they shine).

For those color-blind guys out there: make sure your socks match.

For the ladies: be sure your panty hose or stockings don't have runs.

CHECKLIST

❏ Schedule interviews

❏ Prepare interview wardrobe

NOTES

November Year 1
The Interview Trail: Content Prep

"By failing to prepare, you are preparing to fail."
-BENJAMIN FRANKLIN

Now that your style prep is complete, you can focus on content. The most important content challenge to conquer for medical school interviews is about you. Yes, you likely know yourself well by this point, but you must be able to present this knowledge eloquently to the interviewer. Some people have a very hard time speaking about their own accomplishments. Get over it. You are your only champion at this point in the application. As with everything else in life, becoming a great interviewee takes practice, practice, and practice.

NOVEMBER WEEK 1
Interviews: Why Do You Want to Be a Doctor?

Start your interview prep by answering this question:

"Why do you want to be a doctor?"

Simple, huh? Go ahead and try to answer it right now.

Harder than it seems, isn't it?

This question will be asked in some form in every interview. You answered it in the AMCAS primary essay, but interviewers want to hear it again. It is *the* essential question, right?

The best way to answer the question is clearly and concisely with no more than three talking points. The human brain learns best if points are made in groups of three or less. And tying these three reasons to concise anecdotes will help the interviewer remember your reasons. Here are some examples of effective answers to *the* question:

1. I am drawn to the medical field because it lies at the intersection of art and science. Although staying up-to-date on evidence-based medicine is paramount for every practicing physician, I am equally interested in the story-telling aspect of being a physician. I look forward to listening to my patients' stories and one day sharing these narratives through medical journalism. I have already chronicled my experiences volunteering at the local hospital through a weekly column in my university's newspaper.

2. I want a career that allows me to work with individuals from all walks of life on a daily basis, encourages continual learning, and permits collaboration with other fields including government, business, and information technology. Through speaking with physicians and patients while volunteering at Mercy Hospital HIV Clinic and working as a research assistant at the National Institute, I have come to realize that medicine meets all of these requirements.

3. My passion for medicine comes from a desire to bring cutting-edge laboratory work to the bedside. While working in Dr. Igo Maniac's lab studying the possible uses of RNAi technology to treat Huntington's disease, I have met multiple patients with this devastating illness. I want to help create cures for conditions that are now incurable. By running both a clinic and a basic science laboratory, I believe I can make the biggest contribution to the field.

4. I want to enter medicine so I can become a surgeon who sets up mobile surgical clinics in developing nations. I have spent the last three summers working for Hospital Ships in an administrative role and have witnessed the remarkable impact surgeons can make in underserved areas. I am also drawn to surgery because of its focus on teamwork, use of hand-eye coordination, and opportunity to use advanced technology daily.

NOVEMBER WEEK 2
Interviews: Review AMCAS and Secondary Applications

This week read over the AMCAS and secondary applications for the schools that have offered interviews. Start by reviewing your AMCAS transcript. Every course listed is fair game for the interviewer. You may have taken some of those classes four years ago (or, for some of you, 10 years ago). Take notes on the professor's name, class topic, and the highlight of the class. Now move on to the AMCAS work/activity list. For each activity listed, it is important to remember enough details to answer any question on the topic. Finally, read your personal statement and secondary essays to review the specific information you presented to each school.

To reiterate the importance of this step, I will relay a personal story. While interviewing at Duke, the interviewer asked me what I wanted to do with the "extra" year (Duke squeezes the first two years of medical school into one year so that you have a year to do research or obtain a second degree). I gave what I thought was a great answer about obtaining a MPH. The confused look on the interviewer's face should have tipped me off. Turns out, I wrote my essay on how I would use the free year to continue my study of the history of medicine (my college major). A quick review of my Duke secondary essays would have prevented the mistake.

NOVEMBER WEEK 3
Interviews: Practice, Practice, Practice Questions

Use this week to practice the most typical questions asked in medical school interviews. There are many interview question lists out there on the Internet. Here is the list I give my clients. This is certainly not a comprehensive catalog but is a great starting point. Practice answering these questions out loud in front of a mirror or use your computer/tablet camera to record yourself. You will be surprised by the habits you discover, such as ring twirling, hand wringing, or foot tapping. Practice limiting distracting movements. Also avoid space-fillers such as, "um," "like," and "ya know."

Some applicants like to write down answers to the questions first. This strategy works only if you then practice answering the questions out loud without looking at the written notes. You want to sound polished but not like you are reciting a memorized answer.

Ideally, you should arrange a mock interview with an admissions consultant or medical school counselor. This mock interview should be as close to real as possible. Wear your suit, use an office setting, and answer each question to the best of your ability.

Interview Prep Questions

Most Common Questions
Why do you want to be a doctor?
When did you first become interested in medicine?
What research have you done and why?
How have you served the community?
Where do you see yourself in 10 years?
Why did you choose your undergraduate institution?
Why did you choose your undergraduate major?
What was your favorite college course and why?
How do you know you will enjoy taking care of sick people?
Medicine is a depressing business. How will you cope?
How will you handle the stress of medical school?
If you could not be a doctor, what would you do?
Tell me the most interesting case you have seen.
Why do you want to attend this medical school?
What do you want me to say about you to the admissions committee?
Why should we admit you?

Non-Medical Questions
What is your passion?
What do you do for fun?
What do you do to "blow off steam?"
What is the biggest mistake you have ever made and what did you learn from it?
What are you most proud of that is not on your resume?

What are you most ashamed of?

Who is your idol and why?

Who is your inspiration?

If you were a cereal (animal, book, *etc.*), what kind of cereal would you be?

What is your favorite book (movie, magazine, *etc.*) and why?

If you could have dinner with three people, living or dead, who would they be and why?

Tell me about yourself.

Tell me about your family/upbringing.

Ethics/Policy Questions

What do you think are the biggest challenges facing the healthcare system today?

What are your thoughts on the Affordable Care Act?

What do you think about a public health insurance option?

What do you think about health insurance mandates?

If you were president, what would your health reform bill look like?

What do you think are the three most pressing public health issues facing the United States today?

What do you think of mandating electronic medical records?

How do you feel about euthanasia?

How would you respond to a terminally ill patient requesting help with suicide?

Would you ever perform an abortion? If so, under what circumstances?

What do you think about cloning?

What do you think about pharmaceutical direct advertising to physicians? How about to patients via TV ads?

Would you ever lie to a patient?

If a family member asked you not to tell a patient his diagnosis, what would you do?

Do you think healthcare should be rationed?

Medical mistakes are common but not always important. Significant errors leading to morbidity, such as leaving a sponge in the abdomen after surgery, must be disclosed to patients. Should physicians also disclose less important mistakes, such as a single inconsequential medication error?

Is it acceptable for physicians to modify medical information on insurance forms so companies are more likely to reimburse patients?

How should we deal with "bad" doctors?

A child who is a Jehovah's Witness presents to your hospital after a car accident with an actively bleeding spleen requiring transfusion, and the parents refuse to consent for the child to receive a blood transfusion. What would you do?

A woman with chronic pain and narcotic addiction presents to your office requesting medications. She refuses to leave until you give her narcotics. What do you do?

How do you feel about stem cell research?

The state where you are practicing passes a law requiring you to ask the citizenship status of all your patients and requires you to turn this information into the state at the end of every month. What do you do?

NOVEMBER WEEK 4
Interviews: Current Events

Many interviewers are moving away from standard questions and venturing into questions regarding ethics and current events. During interview season, be sure to stay up-to-date on all current events, especially those related to health care. Read your local paper but also browse national papers such as the *New York Times* and *Washington Post*. *The Economist* politics and business sections provide pertinent and succinct current event reviews. Subscribing to *The Economist* is pricey, but you can read these two sections at the library in less than ten minutes.

CHECKLIST

❑ Prepare answers to most common and difficult interview questions

❑ Practice answering questions in mirror or video record yourself

❑ Review AMCAS and secondary applications

❑ Stay up-to-date on current events

❑ Arrange mock interview

❑ Perform mock interview

NOTES

December Year 1

The Interview Trail: Type, Etiquette, Final Prep, and Notes

"Chance favors only the prepared mind."
-LOUIS PASTEUR

Now that you have mastered your interview style and content preparation, this month focuses on final preparation and interview details that can make or break your interview performance. If you have not arranged for a mock interview yet, this is the time to do so. It is best to do the mock interview about two to three weeks before your first interview to allow time to practice but not providing so much time that you forget what you learned. Given the different types of medical school interviews now used by admissions committees, it may be beneficial for you to undergo multiple mock interview sessions.

DECEMBER WEEK 1
Interviews: Type

Various types of interviews exist on the trail. Most schools use one-on-one "open" interviews where you meet with one interviewer who has read your application. However, "closed" interviews, where the interviewer has not seen your application, are becoming more common. Less common are "semi-open" interviews where the interviewer has read only the personal statement. You will usually meet with two to five interviewers in the interview day. One of the interviewers is often a current medical student at the school. Some schools utilize a group interview for efficiency and to see how you handle a more intimidating situation.

Group interviews can mean either you meet with multiple interviewers at once or you are interviewed with other applicants at the same time. In a group interview when you meet with multiple interviewers at once, address your answer to all the interviewers and not only the person who asked the question. As for interviews where other applicants are involved, try your best not to be intimidated. No matter how the other applicants present themselves, maintain your decorum, never interrupt, and stick to the answers you have practiced.

A new type of interview called the Multiple Mini Interview (MMI) is gaining popularity. Started at McMaster University, MMIs involve multiple short independent questions at different stations, usually in a timed circuit, with each station involving a unique scenario and interviewer. The MMIs focus on an applicant's "soft skills," testing interpersonal relations, moral judgment, teamwork, and professionalism. In general, you will walk up to a room with a written scenario posted on the door. After reading the scenario and taking a moment to think, you will enter the room and do what is asked in the scenario. The entire station generally takes eight to ten minutes. Don't be surprised if there is an actor in the room, you are asked to work with another applicant to solve a problem, or you have to write an essay on the spot. The key to succeeding in MMI interviews is to stick to your personal beliefs, be honest with the interviewer, and not let anyone fluster you.

Here are some MMI question examples:

1. If you caught your friend cheating on an important test, but the professor did not notice, what would you do?

2. Dr. Lee often recommends homeopathic medicines to his patients, even though no scientific evidence exists to suggest homeopathic medicines work, and Dr. Lee does not believe they work. He recommends such medications to patients with mild and non-specific symptoms, such as muscle aches, fatigue, and headaches, because he believes the medicine will do them no harm and will provide reassurance. Consider the ethical problems that Dr. Lee's behavior might pose and discuss these issues with the interviewer.

3. The parking garage at your workplace has assigned parking spots. On leaving your spot, you are observed by the garage attendant as you back out and hit a neighboring BMW, knocking out its left front

headlight and denting the fender. The garage attendant gives you the name and office number of the car owner and then calls ahead to the owner, Tim. The garage attendant tells you Tim is expecting your visit. Enter Tim's office.

Given the wide range of interviewing options, it is best to check with each school ahead of time to know what kind of interview to expect and to direct your mock interviewers on how to best prepare you.

DECEMBER WEEK 2
Interviews: Etiquette

I am sure these tips will seem obvious to you, but you would be surprised by the inappropriate behavior of some applicants. During an interview, avoid:

1. Chewing gum
2. Swearing
3. Using racial slurs
4. Speaking in slang
5. Ticking anybody off

Be as respectful of the receptionist as you are of the interviewers. Rude behavior directed to any of the medical school staff often gets back to the admissions committee and has been known to sink even exceptional candidates.

DECEMBER WEEK 3
Interviews: Final Prep

You have polished your shoes, reviewed your application, and practiced and practiced and practiced questions. Before you leave for an interview, remember these final details:

1. Pack all clothes in a carry-on. I learned the value of this tip the hard way. I didn't show up in jeans to an important interview but came darn close. Airlines lose baggage frequently. Always carry on your luggage.

2. Be sure you have all directions, including public transit options, mapped out. Being late to a medical school interview is not an option.

3. Bring:

   a. Copies of all your publications in case the interviewer would like to see them. You can keep the copies safe in the pocket of a leather legal pad. Then use the legal pad to take notes after the interview.

   b. Blank thank you notes with envelopes and stamps

   c. A snack

   d. Extra pantyhose/stockings in case of runs

   e. Dental floss (very handy for post-lunch interviews)

   f. Cash (always good to have on hand in case of emergency)

4. Ensure a good night's sleep not only the night before, but also the night before the night before the interview. Studies have shown the night previous to the night before is the most important night of sleep for excellent performance in any activity.

DECEMBER WEEK 4
Interviews: Notes

Everyone seems to bring a leather legal pad to interviews. But have you ever seen someone actually taking notes? There is no need to take notes during the interview, as that may seem pretentious. But definitely jot down your thoughts after each interview making special note of:

Interview date

Interviewer name and title spelled correctly

Topics discussed

School positives

School negatives

Overall gut reaction

Taking five minutes to log your thoughts will be helpful in keeping the details of each school straight in your mind and remembering specifics to put in thank you notes.

CHECKLIST

❑ Determine interview type at each school

❑ Complete final interview prep:

    ❑ Pack clothes in carry on bag

    ❑ Obtain directions

    ❑ Bring publication copies, thank you notes, snack, extra stockings, dental floss, and cash

❑ Take notes after each interview

NOTES

January Year 2
Post-Interview Strategy

*"However beautiful the strategy, you
should occasionally look at the results."*
-Sir Winston Churchill

Even after your interviews, there is still more work to be done to gain admission to medical school. Strategically communicating with schools after the interview may increase your chances of acceptance. Well-written thank you notes, update letters, and a letter of intent may effectively remind medical school admission committees why you will be a great asset to their school. Be very careful when using these strategies as one misstep or inappropriate communication can turn an acceptance into a rejection.

JANUARY WEEK 1
Post-Interviews: Thank You Notes

Thank you notes often raise many questions for medical school applicants:

- Do I have to write thank you notes to every interviewer?
- Should the notes be hand-written?
- Will an e-mail serve as a sufficient thank you?

I advise that you write a hand-written thank you note to every interviewer at any school you might attend if accepted. Thank you notes are a priceless way to remind the interviewer of who you are and why you should be accepted. Such an important communication should not be sent to someone's already full e-mail inbox. Writing thank you notes seems like a lot of work, right? It is not. Here are some tricks:

1. Bring thank you notes, envelopes, and stamps with you on the interview.
2. After every interview, note the interviewer's name/title and the most interesting topics you discussed. Be sure to get the exact spelling of each interviewer's name.
3. While traveling home by plane, train, *etc.,* write the thank you notes and then drop them in the mail immediately. If you travel by car, write them before you leave. Delaying thank you notes until "later" means they will never get done. And it is always best to write them while the interview is still fresh in your mind. You will be shocked how interviews can run together on the trail.

Here's an example of a good thank you note:

Dear Dr. Miller,

It was a pleasure to meet you on December 17 and hear about the innovative problem-based learning curriculum and cutting-edge research opportunities at Man's Greatest Medical School. I especially appreciate your interest in my recent study on marathon running and its effect on cardiovascular health and will certainly update you when the manuscript is accepted for publication. I also enjoyed talking about the recent success of the DC University basketball team, and I hope you will see us in the NCAA tournament again this year. Have a wonderful holiday.

Sincerely,

Jane Doe

As you can see in this thank you note example, you want to:
1. Spell the interviewer's name correctly and use the appropriate prefix
2. Remind the interviewer of the interview date

3. Express specific interest in the school in areas such as:
    a. Curriculum type
    b. Research
    c. Community service
    d. Clinical opportunities
    e. Location
4. Highlight your strengths and unique characteristics discussed in the interview in areas such as:
    a. Research
    b. Community service
    c. Athletics/arts/extracurriculars
    d. Clinical experience
5. Close with a cordial statement

Happy writing!

JANUARY WEEK 2
Post-Interviews: Letter of Intent/Update Letters

Some rolling admissions schools have already given you their decision. You may be on waitlists or you have not heard from other schools. This time of year, the question often arises, "Do I tell my top choice it is my top choice?"

The answer is, "Yes."

If you have an absolute top choice and have not been accepted, writing a "letter of intent" may improve your chances of acceptance. Medical schools want students who want them. You may tell only one school it is "the one," so be sure it really is your top choice.

Write a letter to the dean of admissions explaining why the school is your top choice. Include specifics on curriculum, research opportunities, location, *etc.* and reiterate your strengths. This should be a formal yet short letter, ideally less than a page. Send the letter both by regular mail and e-mail to ensure it is received.

Here's an outline to guide the writing of your letter of intent or update letters:

- Formal letter opening with your address, date, recipient address, and salutation.
- Paragraph I: Open with reason for writing. If writing a letter of intent, be sure to state the school is your top choice and you would attend if accepted.
- Paragraph II: Provide update(s) if any exist
- Paragraph III: Discuss why you are a good fit for the school. Be specific. You can merge the II and III paragraphs if your updates lend themselves to explaining why you are a good fit for the school.
- Paragraph IV: Discuss why the school is a good fit for you. Again, be specific.
- Close with sign off, formal salutation, and your signature with printed name

Many medical school applicants ask if they may send a letter of intent to multiple schools. By strict definition, a letter of intent should be sent only to your top choice. However, you can send an "update letter" to your top five or ten schools. Such a letter will follow a similar format to the letter of intent but will not state outright that the school is your top choice and will focus more on updating your recent progress. For example, such updates may include a recent publication, new grades from a post-baccalaureate program, an international experience from the fall, or a new leadership position. These letters should also be formal in style and kept to less than a page.

Also keep in mind that a few schools have "no contact" policies, usually for waitlist applicants. Schools with this policy take it very seriously. Do not call, e-mail, or write letters. Don't have a friend of a friend make a call on your behalf. Take the no contact policy literally. If you would like to be moved from the waitlist to the rejected list, feel free to give the school a call.

Please see letter of intent/update letter examples in Appendix IV.

JANUARY WEEK 3
Post-Interviews: More Recommendations

Many clients come to me for help formulating a waitlist strategy. After writing a letter of intent to the top choice school and update letters to another five to ten schools, clients often ask if calls from recommenders or school alumni to the admissions office are beneficial. In general, any glowing recommendations will help your case. But calls should come only from recommenders who know you well. A call from your uncle's cousin's wife who has met you once but happened to graduate from your waitlisted school will not be of much help and might even hurt you. So be smart. A glowing phone call or an unsolicited written recommendation may improve your application, but don't inundate the admissions staff with calls or letters.

JANUARY WEEK 4
Post-Interviews: Best Behavior

This is the time of medical school admissions decisions. You likely have heard and will continue to hear from schools regarding your interview and acceptance status. Every school has a different timeline for reviewing applications and offering interviews and acceptances. Naturally, you may feel inclined to check in with certain schools to see when final decisions will be made. Even though this is a time of high anxiety, please be sure to be polite when contacting schools. Angering the assistant answering the phone is a very easy way to lose any chance of acceptance. Also, remember to avoid slang, acronyms, and text shorthand in e-mails to schools. Use formal language in all phone calls and e-mail messages.

CHECKLIST

❑ Write thank you notes

❑ Compose letter of intent to top choice school

❑ Write update letters to five to ten other schools

NOTES

February Year 2

Medical School Admissions Limbo

"I'd rather be a 'could-be', if I cannot be an 'are;' because a 'could-be' is a 'maybe' who is reaching for a star. I'd rather be a 'has-been' than a 'might-have-been,' by far; for a 'might-have-been' has never 'been,' but a 'has' was once an 'are.'"
-Milton Berle

February is an odd time in the admissions process. Some schools have already filled their classes while others are still interviewing and have offered no acceptances. During this limbo period, take stock of your situation. Have you not received an interview? If so, it's time to start making phone calls. Overwhelmed with interviews and already have an acceptance? Think about canceling some interviews. Not accepted yet? Focus on the post-interview strategies provided in the January Year 2 chapter. As you now well know, the medical school admission process is both physically and emotionally challenging. Brace yourself for rejections. They likely have and will start arriving. But remember, it only takes one acceptance for you to become a doctor.

FEBRUARY WEEK 1
Admissions Limbo: No Interviews Yet?

Are you still waiting for a medical school interview invite? If so, it is time to get to work. Here are some suggestions:

1. Call each school where you have applied and returned a secondary application. Ask if your application is complete. Also ask if all interview invitations have been given. If the answer is yes, consider this a rejection.
2. Call each school where you have not received a secondary and ensure the school has everything it needs prior to sending a secondary application. Also inquire whether more secondaries will be sent out (quite unlikely at this stage in the interview process, but it does not hurt to ask).
3. Contact your undergraduate or post-baccalaureate pre-med advisor and update him or her on your situation. Some pre-med advisors will make a call on your behalf if a particular school you are interested in attending has not yet offered an interview.

If you obtain an interview at this late stage, congratulations! Be sure to review the interview preparation and post-interview strategy information provided in the October Year 1 to January Year 2 chapters.

If you have performed the three strategies above and still do not receive any interviews, you will likely not be accepted during this admissions cycle. This can be very difficult news to hear but does not mean you will never become a physician. You are allowed to reapply to medical school. Take this time to analyze your application. Why do you think you did not receive an interview? What weaknesses in your application can be improved? Once you have identified the holes in your application, you can start deciding how to fix them. With the next admissions cycle accepting applications in just four months, now is the time to decide how to increase your chances of admission when reapplying. I strongly suggest speaking to an admissions expert, such as your school's pre-med advisor or a private admissions consultant, to obtain an objective opinion and strategize the next steps. Reapplicant strategies are discussed in Appendix V.

FEBRUARY WEEK 2
Admissions Limbo: Avoid Interview Burnout

The time and energy required for medical school interviews can be taxing. Are you one of the few who have more interviews than you know what to do with?

Are you finding school or work slipping because you are always flying off to an interview? Do you think your performance in interviews is sub-par because of fatigue? If so, you should be very grateful. And you should also think about canceling some of the interviews to avoid burnout. Look at the list of interviews you have left. Only attend interviews at schools you will seriously consider attending if accepted. For example, you have already been accepted to one of your top choices and have a few "safety school" interviews in February. Do yourself and the admissions committees a favor and call to cancel those interviews. Also think of those who have not yet received interviews. Your cancellation may open a spot for another applicant. There are no awards given to those who receive the most medical school admission offers.

FEBRUARY WEEK 3
Admissions Limbo: Interview Season Winding Down

Most schools wind down the interview season in late February. If you have not received an interview invitation from a school at this point, you can consider that a rejection. Many schools, unfortunately, will never officially contact you to provide a rejection.

Focus your energies on schools where you have been interviewed and either are waiting to hear about your admissions status or have been waitlisted. Write a letter of intent to your top choice or update letters to other schools of interest to you. Please return to the January chapter for specifics on post-interview strategy including how to write a letter of intent and update letters.

This stage of the medical school admissions process is often a painful waiting game. It can be very difficult. Hang in there.

FEBRUARY WEEK 4
Admissions Limbo: It's Not Personal

With the interview season winding down, the admissions committees are starting to make their final decisions. You have probably heard from rolling admission schools. Most non-rolling admission schools start to extend offers in late February and early March.

Many applicants to medical school are used to doing well in whatever they put their minds to—be it academics, extracurriculars, or research. One of the hardest parts of the medical school admissions process is being rejected. Remember that being denied admission to your favorite medical school has no bearing on your self-worth. It also does not mean you will not be accepted elsewhere. Though admissions committees do not like to admit it, there is significant luck involved in the process. What if the person in charge of reading your AMCAS application had a bad day and didn't give your essay full attention? What if your interviewer did not stay in the committee meeting to push for your acceptance and instead only filled out the standard evaluation sheet? What if three stellar candidates with your same major and similar non-academic experience all applied to the same school? When you look at all the steps involved in acceptance to medical school, it is amazing that anyone gets in at all. If you receive a rejection, don't despair. Resolve to do your best with other opportunities.

CHECKLIST

❑ Contact schools that have not sent secondaries or interview invitations

❑ Call undergraduate pre-med advisor and/or admissions consultant to discuss strategy

❑ Cancel interviews to avoid burnout

NOTES

March Year 2
Acceptances, Rejections, and Waitlists, Oh My!

"Uncertainty is the only certainty there is, and knowing how to live with insecurity is the only security."
-JOHN ALLEN PAULOS

March, like February, is another month filled with significant waiting. Fortunately, most schools will finally make their acceptance offers in March. But with acceptances also come waitlists, holds, deferrals, and rejections. The vocabulary can be confusing, but it is important to understand medical school admissions lingo.

MARCH WEEK 1
Admissions Limbo: Multiple Acceptances

By early March, you likely will have heard from schools regarding your acceptance, waitlist, or rejection status. Many schools put a strict deadline on responding to the acceptance, meaning you will have to accept or decline the offer within a certain period of time. Fortunately, you may hold multiple acceptances and defer your final decision until May 15. On May 15, you must withdraw your acceptance to all but one school.

Though it may boost your ego to hold multiple acceptances, please say yes only to schools you are seriously considering. Do not confirm multiple acceptances just so you can brag on Student Doctor Network. Try to make a decision early so others can get off the waitlist.

MARCH WEEK 2
Admissions Limbo: What the Heck is a Hold?

Back in the old days, medical school admissions were simple. You were either accepted, rejected, or waitlisted. To complicate the already harried lives of medical school applicants, some schools have invented other categories, such as "hold," "alternate," and "deferred." These words have various meanings depending on the school. At some schools, a hold is a better designation than a waitlist. At others, a hold means your application is put in a pool to be evaluated again. Still other schools consider a hold equivalent to a rejection. If you receive one of these less straightforward designations, call the admissions office and ask for a definition.

MARCH WEEK 3
Admissions Limbo: March 15 Deadline

By March 15, all AMCAS schools are supposed to have offered the same number of acceptances as spaces available for that year. But this does not mean that the schools have to tell you about waitlist or rejection status. Some schools will not confirm your status until April and others will never contact you. Check the website of each school for information to see when it offers acceptances. If the website does not have the information, call the admissions office. Be sure to be polite to the person answering the phone.

MARCH WEEK 4
Admissions Limbo: Deferral

"Deferral" refers to the act of a student postponing medical school for one year but holding an admissions spot at a specific school. Deferral is an excellent option if you have an academic fellowship, amazing international opportunity, or want to finish a research project prior to starting medical school. Most schools do not hand out deferrals lightly and request a specific explanation for taking the year "off." In addition, most schools do not allow you to apply again during the deferral period. So you cannot defer a spot at a less prestigious school in order to try again at your top choice. Also, do not advertise that you wish to seek a deferral until you have received an acceptance at a specific school. Schools prefer you apply during the cycle prior to matriculation.

Once you are accepted, call the admissions office and ask for information on the deferral process. You can also look on each school's website as deferral policies are often listed. For example, Harvard Medical School lists its deferral policy on their website:

> Accepted students who would like to apply for deferral must write to the Faculty Associate Dean for Admissions stating their reason for requesting deferral and their proposed plans for the duration of the deferral. We cannot guarantee deferral requests will be granted. If approved, the deferral is typically granted for one year, though they are routinely renewed for students involved in multi-year fellowship programs. The Committee on Admissions is generally supportive of proposals that provide for participation in intellectually rewarding opportunities and service programs during the time of deferral from HMS. (http://hms.harvard.edu/departments/admissions/applying/application-process-and-timeline/deferred-admissions).

University of California San Francisco Medical School states its deferment policy as:

> In special circumstances, the Executive Board for the Committee on Admissions will review requests for deferred admission. Written requests for deferral must be received by May 1 of the year of expected entry. We typically consider deferrals that permit applicants to participate in time-limited, once-in-a-lifetime academic opportunities that will significantly enhance their medical education and training. While we understand that students may wish to spend a year between undergraduate college and the rigors of medical school for financial reasons, personal development, or family needs, we are unlikely to grant deferrals for these reasons. (http://meded.ucsf.edu/admissions/accepted).

Do not assume you will be able to defer. Private schools tend to be more lenient but deferral is never guaranteed. But do know the option is available. Pay attention to deadlines as some schools want to know if you will defer even before the May 15 deadline for holding only one acceptance.

Whether to defer or not is another question. Many applicants feel urgency to start medical school as soon as possible given the length of medical school, residency, and fellowship training. They worry that deferring for a year will make them less competitive medical students and lengthen the time before earning an attending physician salary. I argue that taking one year to pursue an incredible opportunity is priceless. It is difficult to get off the medical roller-coaster as it winds from one training program to another. Family obligations and time commitments only increase with age. If you have a once-in-a-lifetime opportunity, do it and do it now.

CHECKLIST

❑ Meet acceptance offer deadlines

❑ Only hold acceptances at schools you likely will attend

❑ Contact schools to clarify "hold," "alternate," and "deferred" status

❑ Apply for deferral if desired

NOTES

April Year 2
Medical School Choice: Decision Time

"When you approach a problem, strip yourself of preconceived opinions and prejudice, assemble and learn the facts of the situation, make the decision which seems to you to be the most honest, and then stick to it."
-CHESTER BOWLES

April has arrived and many of you have received one or more acceptances to medical school. Congratulations! With the thrill of multiple acceptances comes choice. April is the time to decide where you are going to become a doctor.

For those of you still on the waitlist or waiting to hear from schools, re-read the post-interview strategy in the January Year 2 chapter and consider contacting an admissions consultant for help.

APRIL WEEK 1
Medical School Choice: Location, Location, Location

Multiple factors should guide you in choosing which medical school to attend. Location is paramount. You will be living in this place for at least the next four years. Do you like the city/town? Do you have family, friends, or other social supports nearby? How is the weather? Is there anything to do outside of medicine? Does the location support your extracurricular and community service goals? Can you afford to live there?

As real estate agents always say, "Location, location, location." Location is just as important when deciding on a medical school. Choose wisely.

APRIL WEEK 2
Medical School Choice: People

Still trying to decide which medical school to attend? Along with location, people are a top priority.

Did you like the students, professors, and administrators you met on the interview day? Did they seem happy, stressed, well rounded, nerdy, delinquent, down-to-earth, competitive, genuine, callous, service oriented, *etc.*? Do you fit in at this medical school? Would you enjoy doing a group project with the students you met? Medical school happiness is often based on the people who surround you. Be sure you like them.

Unsure about the people at a certain school? Call and ask the admissions office if there are students you can talk to on the phone. Ask your medical school advisor if any alumni from your undergraduate institution attended the school and contact them. Ask your family members if they know anyone who went to the school. Ask around. You will glean significant information by talking with current and previous students about their experiences.

APRIL 15 DEADLINE

If you are looking to attend a school whose first day of class is on or before July 30, you must make your final decision by April 15. This means that by April 15 you must have informed your top choice that you are accepting the acceptance offer and withdrawn your application from all other schools where you hold an acceptance. For schools beginning class after July 30, the deadline is May 15 to make your final decision.

APRIL WEEK 3
Medical School Choice: Curriculum

For the past couple of weeks, we have been discussing how to choose a medical school. Location and people top the list. The curriculum is another important criterion to think about.

How do you learn? Do you prefer formal lectures or small group learning? Do you learn better on your own or with study partners? Are you motivated by grades or do you prefer a "pass-fail" environment? Though the trend in medical school education is toward "problem-based learning" in small groups, some schools still focus on the more traditional lecture method. Be honest with yourself about how you best learn (it is ok if you like traditional lectures better than small-group learning) and choose a school whose curriculum fits your learning style.

Don't be fooled by "pass-fail" schools offering high pass, pass, and fail. That is basically an A, B, and F grading system and creates competition for those few A slots. If you want a less competitive, truly pass-fail environment, confirm the exact evaluation system for each institution. Schools often have grading systems in the first two years that differ from the last two years. Be sure you are informed.

APRIL WEEK 4
Medical School Choice: Financial Aid

When deciding which school to attend, money will likely play a role. Beyond the obvious tuition and fee expenses, research the following:

What are the living expenses (rent, food, gas, medical insurance)?

Does the school provide subsidized housing?

Do you need a car?

Can you take a 5th year to do research or travel without paying extra tuition?

Are resident advisor positions that provide free room and board on campus available in return for some service to the school?

Does the curriculum allow any time to hold a part-time job?

What financial aid options are available?

Do you have interest in joining the military or public service corps so the government pays?

You may not believe it, but Harvard Medical School was my least expensive private school option because:

1. I didn't need a car.
2. I lived and dined for free as a resident tutor for four years.

Remember, the Free Application for Federal Student Aid (FAFSA, http://www.fafsa.ed.gov/) is due June 30. It is best to turn in the FAFSA forms as early as possible so you will know your financial aid options early. Each school uses the FAFSA along with its own criteria to determine your financial aid package. You may be surprised how the value of these packages can vary by school. If your top choice school offers a less beneficial financial aid package than other schools, you should bring this up with the school's financial aid office. Many times, the packages are adjustable. Also, some medical schools have scholarships based on academic success, gender, or disadvantaged status. Ask each admissions office if scholarships exist.

CHECKLIST

❑ Weigh pros and cons of each school where accepted

❑ Fill out FAFSA and school financial aid forms

NOTES

May Year 2
Medical School Choice:
Really Decision Time

*"Take time to deliberate, but when the time for
action has arrived, stop thinking and go in."*
- NAPOLEON BONAPARTE

With the May 15 deadline fast approaching, it is nearly time to make the final decision about where you will be attending medical school. This month reviews a few more important areas to look at as you weigh the options.

MAY WEEK 1
Medical School Choice: Residency Success

We have already discussed the importance of location, people, curriculum, and cost in making your decision. Another less obvious area to look at is residency success.

Where and in what fields do the students match for residency? Each medical school should have a residency match list readily available and it can often be found on the website. If not, call the admissions office and ask the see the school's "match list" for the past few years. This will give you an excellent sense of whether medical students from each school are going into areas of medicine and residency programs where you have an interest.

Do not be surprised that the majority of students match at the home institution or in the same geographic area. People tend to stay close to where they go to school. This is another reason why location is so important.

MAY WEEK 2
Medical School Choice: Extracurricular, Community Service, and Research Options

The final decision deadline is upon us. Here are a few other specifics to look into when making your medical school choice—extracurricular, community service, and research options. Remember, medical school is not all about academics. You want to stay well rounded, just as you did in college. Does the school support your love of swimming? Are there any community service options that interest you? Do potential mentors exist in your research area? What about international opportunities? Think about what you do to relieve stress and keep yourself happy. Will you be able to continue these activities in the medical schools you are considering?

MAY WEEK 3
Medical School Choice: May 15th Deadline

The day has arrived. By May 15, each applicant who has received an acceptance offer from more than one school must choose where he or she wishes to attend and withdraw applications from all other schools. Check with each school to determine how it wants to be informed. Some require written correspondence by regular mail while others will accept an e-mail notification.

Making a last-minute decision? In the end, you can make a hundred pro-con lists but the decision should come down to gut. Where do you feel the most comfortable? Where do you really want to train to become a doctor and spend the next (at least) four years of your life? I'll bet deep down you know. Decide now.

After May 15, many schools start making offers to those on the waitlist, as applicants are no longer able to hold multiple acceptances. So if you are stuck on the waitlist, you may start hearing from schools soon. Waitlists stay open until the day before school begins in the fall. While waiting, review the post-interview strategies discussed in the January Year 2 chapter and the reapplication strategies laid out in Appendix V.

CHECKLIST

❑ Decide where to attend medical school

❑ Withdraw acceptances to all but one school

❑ Celebrate!

NOTES

Appendix I
AMCAS Personal Statement Examples

I t is always helpful to see examples of successful personal statements to trigger your own creative process. Please notice how no one formula exists when writing a great personal statement. Styles vary dramatically. And that is the point. Personal statements are supposed to be, well, personal. Everyone has a different story to tell. Which means that everyone, including you, can write a unique and compelling essay.

These examples are included only as examples. There is no need to copy the essays' styles, as your goal is to write in your own voice and tell your own story. In other words, please don't plagiarize.

Also note that all names, dates, and personal information have been removed or changed in these essays to protect the authors' privacy. These changes lead to generalized statements, such as "in the Caribbean" or "a university." When writing your personal statement, you, of course, want to be as specific as possible.

PERSONAL STATEMENT EXAMPLE 1
Anecdotes

The author of the following essay is passionate about global health. Instead of simply stating this fact, however, he makes his passion come alive through anecdotes. After reading this essay, you definitely appreciate the author's dedication to caring for the underserved global population. But you also remember Dr. Hernandez, Sanjukta, and water filters in the Caribbean. In a stack of hundreds of personal statements, this essay stands out because of the creative use of anecdotes.

How do we transcend barriers? Barriers separate all aspects of our world, from the tangible net dividing players across a tennis court to the more intangible barricades that segregated races in apartheid South Africa. Their effects range from shaping the foundation of a sport to perpetuating an egregious cultural hegemony. My first memorable encounter with barriers in a medical context emerged when I translated in a rural Central American free clinic. Seemingly routine encounters were plagued with barriers between doctors and underserved patients resulting in substandard care.

At the clinic, I quickly noticed that volunteer physicians almost uniformly relied on the uneducated patients to articulate their own medical needs without probing further. The patients, relying on trusted neighbors for medical advice, usually requested vitamins to cure all ills. Most physicians approved the requests to satisfy the patients. Dr. Hernandez proceeded differently.

An elderly woman entered with her daughter. Her feet festered with an infection untreated for 14 years. Despite Dr. Hernandez's concern, the patient insisted on vitamins. Though a clash of expectations about healthcare delivery separated Dr. Hernandez and his patient, he did not follow the easy path and merely honor the patient's request. Instead, with gentle education of both the patient and her daughter, he helped them understand the importance of antibiotics and surgery to treat the infection. With an appetite to explore the power of communication in knocking down such obstacles as Dr. Hernandez did in Central America, I undertook an AIDS awareness project in India.

My work in four Indian slums brought me into contact with many impoverished individuals. Among them was Sanjukta, a girl whose eyes emanated such a palpable sense of despair that I immediately felt compelled to help her. Sanjukta had neglected her anti-AIDS medicine, seeing no value in taking it. Since the health workers could not dedicate resources to ensure her compliance, I decided to offer what I could give to Sanjukta: my time.

Knowing Sanjukta could be ostracized if her neighbors discovered she had AIDS, we met away from her home. Learning that her husband had deceived her about his HIV-positive status, I was not surprised to find Sanjukta guarded. Looking to build trust through communication, I found a connection through our common interest in languages. Sanjukta began sharing how AIDS had left her with little energy and such dejection that she gave up teaching Hindi to children in the local slum school, her biggest joy. As I reasoned that by taking medicine she could renew her energy and resume teaching, her outlook seemed to change.

Only weeks later, Sanjukta's smile revealed new hope. Following her medication regimen, she had returned to teaching. Sanjukta's improvement revealed the potential of personal connection to transcend cultural barriers. However, my impact depended on medical science to extend her life. Recognizing the power of combining culturally-sensitive communication and modern science in one patient's life fueled my desire to utilize this hybrid to improve health on a larger scale. I initiated a project in the Caribbean to implement this idea.

Concerned that mountainous villages in the Caribbean lacked access to potable water, I lead a team to assess household conditions to lower the incidence of water-borne illness. Before administering the surveys, we built rapport with the families and became acquainted with their cultural values. From this relationship with the villagers, we discovered their definition of safe water involved water clarity. Using photos of microbes found in transparent water, we convinced the villagers that clear water could still be contaminated. A follow-up conversation on water safety and filtration prompted over 99% of the families to accept the water filters offered. Establishing a connection was pivotal to conveying scientific information within the framework of the villagers' understanding and culture. Coupling thoughtful interaction with scientific research allowed us to make a tangible difference in the health of many families.

Whether navigating around patient misconceptions or negotiating with a patient to take her life-saving medication, my interactions and decisions as a physician will reflect a respect for differing values. As a medical student, I am eager to cultivate the scientific basis for medical practice through formal study as I continue to hone the interpersonal art. By eventually implementing my perspective to promote health domestically and internationally, I hope to assist the medical profession in accomplishing the ultimate goal of shattering all barriers preventing effective healthcare delivery.

PERSONAL STATEMENT EXAMPLE 2
Metaphors

Great authors often use metaphor to make an essay more memorable and cohesive. The following author intertwines a light-hearted metaphor with a heart-wrenching discussion of her mother's illness. She presents an excellent argument as to why she wants to be a physician and, by appropriately using metaphor, stands out.

As a kid, family and friends always teased me for having small feet. My mom told me that her mother wore a size six shoe her entire adult life, so I figured I was doomed to the same fate. While everyone else in my sixth grade class graduated to adult sizes, I still shopped in the kids' section. As I got older and barely grew into the smallest adult shoe size, I noticed something while shopping with my older sister. She wears a size eight, and stores always seem to be sold out of shoes in her size. I, on the other hand, can almost always find my size. I started to think that maybe my small feet weren't such a misfortune.

While trying on shoes can be fun and adventurous, it can also be distressing. February of my freshman year of college, my mother was diagnosed with a degenerative neurological disease called Multiple System Atrophy. She suffers from deterioration of many autonomic functions due to failure of her excretory, circulatory, and nervous systems. Her cerebellum is also deteriorating, causing increasing loss of balance, hand-eye coordination, and speech. The prognosis, steady deterioration for seven to nine years followed by death, has put me in the most difficult and uncomfortable situation. My mom is my voice of reason, my source of advice, and my best friend. My first questions after hearing the prognosis were who I would shop for a wedding dress with, who I would ask advice on child rearing, who I would call at three in the morning when I had a fight with a friend? My mom somehow seems to have the right answers, and I'm not ready to lose that source of wisdom. I'm not ready to wear the shoes of a motherless child, nor am I ready to try on shoes without her by my side.

Despite my lack of readiness, I have no choice but to be flexible and do my best to prepare for wearing these shoes every day for the rest of my life. The best way I found to approach this uncertain time was to embrace it. While I spent the past four years developing my skills as a student and active member of a college community, I also talked to my mom several times each day and told her about my friends, classes, and sports. Whenever I came home, I took my mom to the movies, shopping, and to do errands to break up the monotony of a life lived primarily in one room.

Somewhere between struggling to lift my mother's 200-pound scooter out of the trunk of my car, pardoning her as she bumped into strangers, and driving home from Williamsburg at midnight to meet her in the emergency department, I realized my true calling in life is to care for people. Throughout college, as my goal of becoming a doctor became clearer, I increasingly took the initiative to further my education by conducting independent research in an organic chemistry lab, taking classes such as medical sociology to see the world of medicine through a different lens, and stepping out of my comfort zone to defend an honors thesis to a panel of professors.

In addition to academic endeavors, college provided an opportunity to grow as a leader and volunteer. I participated in READ, a community service program that organizes weekly visits to patients suffering from Alzheimer's disease and dementia. During my sophomore year, I initiated a new program site in order to reach more patients. The new site required developing a relationship with the assisted living facility on behalf of my university, collaboration with the activities coordinator, and hunting for new activities we could perform each week. Keeping a group of fifteen to twenty adults suffering from various stages of mind deterioration focused required originality and patience. I have utilized this ability to adapt to unfamiliar situations and new challenges to better adjust to my mom's illness. While watching her struggle to transfer from one chair to another and listening to her labored breathing patterns, I have devised creative ways to ameliorate the situation. I make games out of tasks, joke to make her smile, and reorganize my work to be portable so I can keep her company.

Witnessing the intense medical care my mom has required and accompanying her on appointments, overnight visits to the emergency room, and week-long stays at an autonomic dysfunction center, I have realized a new curiosity for the human body and an urge to gain the knowledge needed to care for the ill and injured. Through observing doctors who have cared for my mother as well as shadowing physicians in various specialties, I have learned that a good doctor has a firm grasp of medical knowledge. However, great doctors must be able to adapt to new situations, work with anyone who comes in the door, and show the same compassion to each patient that one would show their own mom. Great doctors must possess the ability to try on any shoes the shopkeeper hands them. Whether excelling academically in the classroom and through research, serving Alzheimer's patients, or caring for my mom, I have shown an ability to adapt. I am now ready to wear the shoes of a doctor.

PERSONAL STATEMENT EXAMPLE 3
Creativity

I often cringe when applicants try to be overly creative to stand out. I have seen some major missteps, such as writing the personal statement as a poem or inserting French quotes throughout the essay. The following author, however, utilizes a very unique style that works. When I first learned he wanted to link his life story to his fastest mile time, I worried the essay would sound cliché. But by choosing every word carefully and writing more than ten drafts, this applicant created an excellent and creative personal statement.

My twin-sized, checker-sheeted bed lost any sense of identity as it stood in a row of similarly prepared bunks. Though not technically an orphan, a long and complicated custody battle led this orphanage to serve as my temporary home. When I was going on four, my father left my sister and I in an orphanage and ran off. When people run, often times they finish where they began. Running has played a large role in my life, but I have no intentions of returning to the starting line. Just like obtaining an under five minute 1600-meter time, my race to medicine has involved many hurdles. Overcoming life's challenges, however, has shaped me into an individual that believes pasts do not determine futures and with both kindness and hard work, one can achieve anything.

[0:00] The start: When my stepfather and mother parted ways, I became the man of the house. This is a tall task for any nine year-old but taught me an early lesson in leadership. I matured quickly and learned the importance of hard work and self-reliance. My mother was rarely home, working two jobs whose wages still barely met expenses. Alone at home, I found a way to consume every part of each day. I organized rides to team practices, joined student government, and finished homework on my own.

[1:06] Lap 1: Many people would run the other way if someone offered them a chance to return to high school. I would gladly accept. I had reached an age where I could actively recognize the importance of being a leader. In contrast to my unpredictable life at home, high school provided an environment I could control. I became team captain of the basketball, soccer, and school pep teams, a varsity track runner, and a personal tutor. As captain, I enjoyed finding balance among teaching, challenging, and motivating others. At the end of high school, I earned the Spirit Award from the athletic department and was voted Best Personality and Most Likely To Brighten Your Day by fellow classmates.

[2:18] Lap 2: I spent the summer before college running between three different jobs in order to financially support my pregnant nineteen-year-old sister and to assist in paying the rent and electric bills. Fortunately, earning a position within the Scholars Program at my university covered the cost of college. The scholarship allotted time to volunteer rather than work. I became an active member of Student Ambassadors, as well as a ranked member of several student organizations, a teacher's aide and tutor, and a laboratory research assistant.

[3:31] Lap 3: Senior year in college, I finally got the chance to stretch my legs internationally. Serving as team leader of the Service Learning trip, I helped run clinics for medically underserved areas in Central America. I loved connecting with patients. I fondly remember a young woman who seemed extremely nervous about receiving a tiny prick on her finger for a glucose test. In broken Spanish I told her, "I will not hurt you, but if I hurt you...hit me." While she laughed, I conducted the test without her realizing I stuck her. I found great satisfaction in using humor and interpersonal skills to make patients feel at ease.

[4:56] Lap 4: Running into a trauma bay will always be exciting. Over the past two years, I have worked as lead emergency department scribe at a level I trauma center. As a scribe, I shadow an attending physician while documenting each patient's history and physical exam, placing orders, and anticipating the doctor's needs. Although I have held leadership positions all my life, working as the lead scribe has been challenging. It is an ongoing process of monitoring, adjusting, and then re-evaluating the effectiveness of the training process, communication between physicians and scribes, and electronic medical records. However challenging, this experience has been equally rewarding. I have developed differential forming skills and witnessed the social aspects of medicine. Watching doctors interact with patients, nurses, residents, and medical students has been an ongoing lesson about how to handle different complaints, cultures, and personalities.

Running, like life, has provided a great challenge. Just as I persevered to accomplish my goal of finishing a mile in less than five minutes, I continue to work towards my dream of becoming a physician. I believe my clinical experiences within the emergency department and in Central America, along with my interpersonal skills and work ethic, have shaped me into an individual who is prepared for the academic and social challenges of medicine. I believe my life experiences, highlighted by financial difficulties and family hardships, have shaped me into an individual who is emotionally prepared for the challenge a career in medicine can present. Becoming a physician does not mark the finish line but is the next lap of my personal race.

PERSONAL STATEMENT EXAMPLE 4
Clinical Experiences

Many applicants like to start the personal statement by describing exciting clinical encounters. These anecdotes often sound hollow because the author plays only a passive role. Here is an essay that shows the power of describing active experiences. Even though the clinical anecdotes used are not dramatic in the typical sense, the author's descriptions exude compassion and empathy. After reading this essay, I believe the author will be an excellent listener and caring clinician.

Shifting in his chair, chattering about the warm weather, and avoiding eye contact, the man across from me exuded anxiety. I did not know why Ben had come to a HIV counselor, but I realized direct questioning would not help me find out. I started by addressing the present moment and that he seemed anxious. As we chatted, Ben turned toward me, slowed his speech, and looked me in the eye, revealing that he may have exposed his partner to HIV. After we made a connection and discussed the options, Ben left the counseling session with a cautious resolve to talk frankly with his partner. This counseling interaction exemplifies qualities I will bring to the practice of medicine: the ability to build trust, to respond to people on their own terms, and to see patients as situated in biological, psychological, and cultural contexts.

I learned respect for different cultures from my mother, a school principal who moved us overseas after my father died. While in Central Asia, my mother arranged for a religious ceremony to honor the deity local residents believed lived in trees prior to having a tree removed from school property. Through such actions my mother taught me the importance of interacting with people from other cultures in terms consistent with their worldview.

While my childhood overseas provided invaluable lessons about respecting different cultures, moving almost yearly proved difficult given my natural shyness. I longed to be a real American kid, watching TV and drinking milk from a carton instead of the powdered version in Central Asia and Africa. When we returned to the United States, however, I initially felt lost in American culture. My extreme shyness and sense of dislocation increased in high school and college, leading to social challenges. My academic record reflects my distraction during those years. Despite fitful attempts to finish my degree, I left school to work as a computer programmer, which satisfied my analytic interests but did little to address my isolation.

In the 1990s, the AIDS epidemic refocused my attention on others. Before anti-retroviral combination therapy revolutionized HIV treatment, I cared for several friends dying of AIDS. Though initially terrified of David's thin, ashen body and blind eyes ravaged by CMV, I found a deep sense of peace and clarity helping him maintain his dignity as he became increasingly disabled. Interpreting the wishes of my friend David was difficult because dementia clouded his mind and an esophageal fungal infection inhibited his speech. But with the guidance of his expressive eyes, I learned that small gestures, such as soothing his lips with Vaseline or reading a chapter from Pinocchio, comforted him while he was dying. The opportunity to care for friends triggered self-exploration and led me to successfully obtain help for my own social anxiety.

Healthy and focused, I decided to finish my undergraduate degree. Longing to study new ways of thinking, I majored in philosophy and felt drawn to thinkers who assert that a meaningful life arises from concrete, bodily interaction with other human beings, rather than from isolated, detached reasoning.

To explore connections between body and mind, I volunteered as a research assistant in a Bay Area college's Psychophysiology and Social Interaction Laboratory. There I studied the physiological effects of induced emotions. I also observed dramatic physiological changes in couples during stressful conversations, again demonstrating that an individual's health greatly depends on context—in this case, the context of long-term, intimate relationships.

While finishing school, I reflected upon my satisfaction caring for sick friends, fascination with contextual understanding of human interactions, and lifelong interest in problem solving. I realized that medicine is my calling and immediately set out to gain clinical experience. In addition to working as a HIV counselor, I volunteered as a clinic assistant at an urban community center serving immigrants. There, the trust of a Cantonese teenager who extended her arm for a flu shot reminded me of the fulfillment gained while caring for sick friends. Seeing patients suffer from diabetes because their diet dramatically changed reinforced my sense that health depends on social context. Repeatedly calling social service agencies to help an elderly Guatemalan woman find temporary housing heightened my resolve to use analytic skills to bring systematic change to service delivery and triggered my development of a system that provides clinic patients with health education materials and case management services.

I am drawn to medicine because, uniquely among the care-giving professions, medicine has the ability to address patients as biological, social, and cultural beings. My varied experiences, including growing up overseas, caring for friends dying of AIDS, working as a HIV counselor, and assisting underserved immigrants, have all reinforced that understanding a patient's context is critical to providing appropriate care. As a physician, I will use this knowledge to help people develop their health in accordance with what gives their lives meaning.

PERSONAL STATEMENT EXAMPLE 5
More Clinical Experiences

Clinical experiences are such a common theme in medical school personal statements that I want to provide you with another example. Reading the first few lines of the following personal statement made me groan. Not another "I saved the day" clinical experience personal statement, I thought. But I kept reading and was very pleasantly surprised. The author's unique twist on what could have been a clichéd clinical experience essay makes this personal statement stand out.

"Adult code yellow ETA five minutes by ground." The emergency department loud speaker blared the announcement at the end of my shift. Normally, I would have been headed home, but I wanted to see one final trauma on my last day at the hospital. During the past three-weeks of the Trauma Externship Program, I had been immersed in the drama of a level I trauma center, but I was not ready to let go of the exhilaration I felt when responding to a code. Teeming with anticipation, some part of me hoped this last trauma would be memorable.

While the nurses set up the trauma bay, I learned the background of the incoming code: nineteen year-old female involved in a MVC versus tree. It felt almost anticlimactic; during my limited time at the hospital, I had already witnessed over a dozen patients brought in after car accidents. Still, I waited to see the resulting injuries. As the paramedics entered, I shifted my gaze to assess the patient. While my eyes normally fixated on blood or obvious signs of trauma, I did not notice her multiple lacerations or deformed shoulder. Instead, all I saw were her characteristic chestnut curls springing from the c-collar, her freshly manicured fingers curling over the edge of the yellow backboard, and the familiar scar emerging from just below her jean skirt. I held my breath. She was more than just my last patient; we grew up together and swam on the same swim team for twelve years. She was my friend.

For three-weeks, injuries had overshadowed the identity of patients as I watched physicians and surgeons methodically suture, splint, and cut. But now, rather than treating a wound or a set of symptoms, I witnessed doctors caring for an individual—a daughter, a sister, and my friend. She was comprised of more than medical issues. She had a life and a story I was fortunate to know. For example, the two-inch scar on her right knee was more than a mark; it was a relic of a soccer injury that led to an ACL repair. The jean skirt being cut from her hips was one of her favorites despite the sizeable hole in the back pocket. Because she was more than a patient, I realized the impact of medicine: actualizing possibility for each patient's story.

As a doctor, I will have the opportunity to help my patients advance their lives by improving health. But as my friend lay on the stretcher next to me, I also felt the weight of this responsibility. I had already witnessed the limitations of medicine and the frailty of human life. Having stood by the side of physicians and social workers as they notified families of their losses, I recognized medicine's weaknesses. Yet, I now understood that the fallibility of medicine and the frailty of life make the study of medicine so significant. After all, providing the right medical treatment can mean the difference between continuing a story and concluding one.

With this new appreciation for the humanity of medicine, I used available resources to create opportunities for others. During senior year, I focused my efforts on global health organizations. As an intern for the Global Health Initiative, I dedicated myself to the improvement of maternal health in Africa, fundraising over $85,000 to improve hospital equipment, to provide women with needed procedures, and to train African health professionals in courses such as Neonatal Resuscitation and Advanced Life Support in Obstetrics. I also participated in the foundation of a new student organization that focuses on educating Central American children about health topics such as nutrition, diabetes, hygiene, and self-esteem. As a result of canvassing for the improvement of health conditions in Africa and Central America, I have a unique, global perspective and a greater cultural awareness that I can apply to my work with diverse patient populations.

After focusing my efforts abroad, I find myself back in the emergency department where I once stood observing. Now serving as a medical scribe, I work with physicians to complete medical documentation and enhance patient care. While I still have years before I will practice medicine, my personal experiences have made me realize the responsibilities and possibilities associated with doctoring. This understanding not only drives me to make an impact across the globe, it motivates me to save stories in the future.

PERSONAL STATEMENT EXAMPLE 6
Community Service

Community service is one of the many important criterion medical school admissions committees consider when evaluating an applicant. This essay highlights the applicant's commitment to community service, and then skillfully ties her experiences to overcoming adversity and to her desire to enter medicine.

I met Riley the summer before junior year as part of a buddy program at my university's children's hospital. The similarities she shared with my sister who was also ten struck me. They both enjoyed reading, riding horses, and watching college basketball. However, I soon learned one significant difference between them—Riley had cystic fibrosis. Despite her condition, she acted like an average 10 year-old girl, playing Guitar Hero and drawing cartoons. It wasn't until I saw Riley in physical therapy, wearing a large vest that shook her entire body to break up lung mucus, that I began to see how sick she really was. Before meeting Riley, my desire to practice medicine had been idealistic, unfettered by the realities of pain and hardship. Spending time with Riley in the hospital, performing multiple research projects, and volunteering in New Orleans after Hurricane Katrina showed me that reaching important goals often requires overcoming adversity. I have realized the disparities in quality of life and experience so common in our world and look forward to using hard work and persistence to better the lives of others through medicine.

Persistence has helped me overcome hurdles. During sophomore year, I became overwhelmed with an intensified course load and my grades suffered. The relationship with Riley helped me rebound from this frustrating year, reminding me that hard work and dedication would help me refocus and achieve academic success. Getting to know Riley also drove me to pursue medical research, inspiring investigations that may translate to better bedside care. I began researching deep brain stimulation and its ability to alleviate multiple sclerosis (MS) symptoms. My senior project stemmed from the MS research and focused on improving the biocompatibility in mechanical assistance devices to decrease complications from LVAD surgery. Although the research progressed slowly, watching Riley's and her doctor's consistent determination to fight her disease motivated me to stay focused. Consequently, I re-achieved academic success and completed research that showed seeding cells on titanium ameliorate common complications from LVAD surgery.

My experience in New Orleans also showed me the benefit of persistence and hard work in overcoming adversity. During my freshmen year spring break, I traveled to post-Katrina New Orleans and spent the week clearing houses of sludge and mud. It was exhausting and claustrophobic, but I never forgot the homeowners' smiles and tears. Despite losing everything, they were eager to come back and rebuild a better city. Their determination motivated me to continue helping with the rebuilding process, and I returned to New Orleans as an intern at a local health system. As part of the school district's recovery plan, I helped create an online health career exploration program to educate local students about healthcare. I also assisted with renovation of an elementary school library and tutored math to underserved high school students. The school and the students suffered serious damage from Katrina. Instead of giving up, they showed me perseverance in the face of destruction and hardship.

My academic, research, and community service experiences have shown me the road to recovery is often long and exhausting, but hard work and persistence are powerful tools to overcome obstacles. Riley and her doctors demonstrated unwavering resolve to improve her condition. I saw a renewed dedication to academics and research. New Orleanians showed hope through enthusiasm to rebuild the city. Doctors have their fair share of tragedies and disappointments, but they always pick up the pieces and start anew, motivated to try again. Medicine will give me an outlet to help people down the hard paths in their lives so they, too, can bounce back.

PERSONAL STATEMENT EXAMPLE 7
International Experience

Many applicants have found inspiration participating in international health programs. This author uses her impressive international health experiences as evidence to support her desire to become a physician who serves the under-privileged. Notice the interesting hook. You want to keep reading, right? I certainly did.

"Egbe nkeke nene?" In the West African language, Ewe, this means "for how long?" It was a simple question, but rarely during my time in Africa did I get a straightforward answer. For the unresponsive middle-aged

woman who had suffered a stroke and was wheeled into the clinic, the answer was two weeks. For the elderly woman with an infected foot injury, the answer was sixteen years. For the man with a disfigured foot, a result of an untreated broken ankle, the answer was twenty-four years. Why wait so long before seeking medical treatment? Interestingly, every person's answer was different: no health insurance, not knowing where to go, or simply fear. The delay I witnessed in Africa surely occurs around the world, including in the United States. Although I found observing the consequences and complications of this delay incredibly frustrating, I now understand the reasons for not seeking medical treatment are complex. I realize doctors need to understand not only the physiology of their patients, but also the cultural and social factors that influence the way they seek and receive medical treatment. I believe my unique blend of experiences growing up on three continents, stepping out of my comfort zone when working with children, and volunteering internationally qualifies me to be that kind of doctor.

My life course has revolved around learning how to achieve the goal of providing care to diverse and underserved populations. From an early age, I received an education that helped me become sensitive, tolerant, and open-minded to difference. By the time I was six years old, I had lived on three different continents. My parents, who are from two different countries, raised me to be bilingual in English and Dutch. As a child I moved many times, and as an adult I have chosen to travel to Central Asia and multiple African countries to volunteer. The majority of the experience gained abroad can be applied in the United States.

Throughout my undergraduate education, I stepped out of my comfort zone to acquire medical experience in non-traditional ways. In addition to gaining experiences abroad, I volunteered at a summer camp for children with epilepsy in the Southern US and learned about autism, cerebral palsy, and Tourette's syndrome, as well as how to treat seizures. I also worked in child-care throughout college to help support myself, during which time I learned how to measure blood glucose levels, administer insulin injections, and use an insulin pump. I often pushed myself outside of my comfort zone to discover more about medicine, realizing every time how much satisfaction it brings me.

My experience volunteering in three African countries further convinced me that in order to be an effective physician, it is not sufficient to have a compassionate heart. It is essential to have a cultural understanding of the individuals seeking care. Volunteering in developing countries gave me the opportunity to acquire invaluable, tangible experiences such as standing next to a surgeon in the operating theater, taking patients' vitals, and helping administer HIV tests. It also taught me that many medical professionals can improve their patients' well being through culturally-sensitive education. During a medical outreach in a small African village, I met a fifteen-year-old girl who complained of stomach pains. Ten small square scars covered her abdomen. A translator explained that in her village it is believed a stomachache can be healed by cutting open the abdominal flesh, placing medicine underneath the skin, and waiting for the wound to heal. Education would help appease patients' fears and assist their understanding of how the mechanics of modern medicine can apply to a simple stomachache. I hope to facilitate a better understanding of the benefits of Western science among patients while remaining sensitive to their cultural backgrounds.

My diverse clinical experiences both in the US and abroad have solidified my desire to become a physician. I am confident that I can thrive in the medical field as a bilingual doctor who has experienced multiple cultures from an early age, enjoys stepping out of her comfort zone to learn new tasks, and understands the importance of merging current medical knowledge and cultural sensitivity. Both nationally and internationally, I hope to improve the answer to the simple question, "For how long?"

PERSONAL STATEMENT EXAMPLE 8
Personal Experience with Illness

Many medical school applicants are drawn to healthcare because of personal experiences with illness, whether in themselves or in loved ones. It often can be tricky to discuss personal illnesses without sounding overly dramatic. This author adeptly merges his struggle with cancer into the essay but does not let it weigh down the piece.

Not a week goes by without a news story discussing a link between the environment and health. Carbon emissions, water pollution, ozone depletion, and hazardous wastes have been linked to various cancers and myriad health problems, particularly among the underprivileged. As a former environmental science major and cancer survivor, my deep-seated passion is to understand the connection between the environment and human disease in hopes of finding new ways to prevent and treat such illnesses.

After being named National Hispanic Merit Scholar for my academic performance in high school, I entered college as a presidential scholar and with high hopes for academic success. Diagnosed with lymphoma toward the end of senior year, I started college while still receiving chemotherapy and radiation treatments. Though determined not to let the disease change my life, it certainly affected my academics. Even after chemotherapy concluded, side effects of the drugs including mental fuzziness and memory gaps provided a frustrating obstacle to studying and led me to consider leaving the pre-medical tract. Support of family and the pre-medical counselor helped me stay the course.

After finishing cancer treatment, I gained admission to a pediatric oncology fellowship at the local children's hospital usually reserved for first-year medical students. I attended bi-weekly lectures in all areas of pediatric oncology and weekly tumor board meetings. It quickly became clear that my own experiences with cancer gave me a unique advantage in connecting with patients. Concurrently, I joined a research project at the hospital to determine whether playing cancer-themed video games increased cancer knowledge in children currently under treatment. The research showed that playing the computer game "Re-Mission" increased the children's compliance with medical treatment. As a result, the researchers now aim to develop comparable resources for sickle cell disease, depression, and autism. Whether through lectures, research, or spending time with patients, every moment at the hospital increased my determination to become a physician no matter the obstacles.

Senior year brought another serious challenge. Just prior to fall semester finals, an emergency surgical biopsy confirmed the lymphoma had returned. The relapse forced a leave of absence from college since treatment involved hospitalization for two rounds of intense chemotherapy followed by a stem cell transplant. Once healthy, I put all my effort into continuing medical school preparation. While working part-time as an emergency medical technician to gain more clinical experience, I retook several pre-medical science classes. Proving my ability to excel in science, I earned an A in all courses.

While pursuing academic and clinical interests, I also continued with environmental science research. Through my university, I joined a study abroad research program to assist professors with ongoing research in Central America studying the impact of increased tourism on the country's tropical ecology. A year later, I ventured to an anthropological dig site in Central America to help professors researching environmental factors that may have contributed to the decline of Mayan civilization.

As an environmental researcher and cancer survivor, my main interests lie in pediatrics, oncology, and disease prevention. I have been given a second chance at life and now hope to use education, research, and personal experience to give others that same gift. Further, I hope that understanding the root causes of illness, particularly as related to the environment, can prevent disease from affecting lives altogether.

PERSONAL STATEMENT EXAMPLE 9
Non-traditional Applicant

Non-traditional applicants, defined as those who have taken time off after college before heading to medical school, often struggle to concisely tell their stories given increased life experiences. "How do I boil down 27 years of life into one page?" one of my client's questioned. "My resume is five pages long. I can't condense my life story into 5300 characters," another client bemoaned. It may not be easy, but it is possible.

A 40-year old applicant with extraordinary life experience and a very long resume wrote the following essay. Though a bit longer than I usually suggest, this essay adeptly weaves her many experiences into an intriguing story. The author even gets away with starting with a quote (which I do not recommend), but it works here. She also does an excellent job of creating a strong theme (problem solving) and weaving it throughout the entire essay. Also notice how she subtly yet effectively addresses a poor college academic record.

"Devin, could you invent a vocal part that sounds like a cross between Pink Floyd and K.D. Lang? We need a spectacular finish for the song." I breathed deeply and stepped to the microphone, not yet knowing what to sing. I had first heard this song only an hour before and could feel the songwriter and album producer listening from outside the recording booth. This is just another type of problem to solve, I reminded myself; listen to how the parts fit together and the answer will come. I began to sing, drawing on my decades of musical experience, and wove my voice among the parts to create a new, complete whole.

Problem solving has been a lifelong passion. My parents, a physician and psychologist, fostered my analytic nature by supporting scientific exploration. They even encouraged me to take apart the family piano and figure out how to reassemble it. Surrounded by hundreds of piano parts spread across the living room floor, I was in my element. The satisfaction I felt from successfully fitting each piano piece together equaled my pleasure in learning how the whole worked.

In my senior year of high school, my love of health and science led me to design an award-winning research study comparing Asian and North American attitudes towards employment of the disabled. This time, the puzzle pieces were much more complex and required statistical analysis to fit them together. But I learned that the Asians I surveyed had a more negative attitude towards disabled employment than my subjects in the United States.

In college, I pursued my interest in science by majoring in biological anthropology and exploring the nuts and bolts of physical science. While enjoying classes on physiology and endocrinology, I also worked as machinist for the science department. Designing and building physics lecture demonstrations earned me the title of "Plexi-Queen." Though I loved the science, a newfound passion for creating music led to over-commitments and uncharacteristic academic performance. Yet, as alto and financial officer for my university's a capella group, I learned how to solve a very different set of problems: how to manage a budget, produce a lucrative music tour, and be a creative part of a close-knit team.

After college, my interest in problem solving led to a career in software. I found that the same techniques I used to reassemble the family piano translated well to management. At a software company, my first managerial role involved molding a group of disgruntled employees into a functioning team. Taking the time to listen to each team member allowed me to discern their individual strengths and craft a model that fit them together more effectively. The team soon functioned efficiently and its members expressed increased job satisfaction.

Although working in software has been intellectually stimulating, finding a truly satisfying career has been my biggest challenge. My ideal profession would mesh my love of health and science, the creativity learned from songwriting, and the management skills honed in the software world. I had occasionally considered a medical career but did not sufficiently understand day-to-day physician life. Then, a few years ago, a thrilling introduction to the human body grabbed my attention.

On the first day of Mini Medical School, a neurology professor riveted me with his epileptic seizure imitation and subsequent explanation of how the brain created such movement. Later, I had the privilege of working with a human cadaver. While other students hung back, my gloved hands left no organ unhandled. For the first time, I understood that the human body is one of the most fascinating puzzles of all. Seeing the intricate machinery of the human arm, with its slick, white ribbons of tendon functioning so closely to the other delicate parts of the wrist, sparked an intense investigation of medical careers. After shadowing several doctors and observing surgeries, I entered a post-baccalaureate pre-medical program and delved into multiple volunteer opportunities.

Working closely with patients through volunteering has reinforced my commitment to a medical career. At a local hospital's emergency department, helping roll trauma victims gives me respect for the quick decisions physicians must make in critical situations. Washing the gnarled feet of a homeless woman at a free inner city clinic who could not afford properly fitting shoes showed me how a person's socio-economic status challenges the ability to heal. Laughing with a young man at a health center serving the uninsured who could converse only via a small whiteboard reminded me of the communication challenges physicians face daily. I believe my analytic, creative, and managerial skills will help me be an efficient problem-solver, compassionate clinician, and effective communicator.

Just as I did when finding a new vocal part that day in the recording studio, I have listened to the parts of my life and learned how they can fit together into a rewarding career. I look forward to the day when I can apply my problem solving skills to curing an illness or running a clinic and see my efforts result in the improved health of a patient and community.

PERSONAL STATEMENT EXAMPLE 10
Non-Science Major

You do not need to major in science to become a doctor. In fact, medical schools love humanities majors. I majored in a branch of history. The following essay does a nice job of using the applicant's liberal arts education as a springboard to discuss her creative and multifaceted approach to life and path to medicine. Also notice how the author's discussion of a low MCAT score merges seamlessly into the theme of viewing the world from different angles.

10:16AM. It was the final push. The student midwife stood by Silvia's side while the doctor crouched down, hands on the baby's head, ready to catch as it came tumbling out. As I watched the baby slowly descend, my heart pounded with the anticipation of witnessing a birth for the first time. Sweat dripped down the mother's forehead and, as she breathed deeply, she focused her eyes on mine. "*Respira profundo...otra vez,*" I coaxed between pushes.

I had met Silvia and her husband, José, just a few weeks earlier at a free urban clinic and felt gratified that I had succeeded in gaining the trust of a patient. Like many of our immigrant patients with no insurance or support network, they arrived seeking health care and a sense of community. Working at the clinic has allowed me to put my commitment to equitable healthcare into practice while gaining greater insight into the dynamic interaction of socioeconomic and cultural factors affecting health. An interest in utilizing a multifaceted approach to make a concrete difference in the health of others has guided my academic and extracurricular choices.

I chose a liberal arts undergraduate education to obtain a solid foundation across disciplines. Early in college, I began to weave together the strands of my interests in social justice, health, and art to design an interdisciplinary major. This multifaceted approach likely stemmed from my viewing the world through the unique lens of dyslexia. Diagnosed in elementary school, I developed effective learning strategies and always excelled academically. Paradoxically, my strong academic record led to the denial of time accommodation on the MCAT and a score unreflective of my ability. Yet, as a consequence of the challenges I faced, I learned the value of taking initiative and approaching material from different angles.

The benefits of a multifaceted approach to problem solving became even more apparent during research abroad and senior thesis work. Entering the world of global health illustrated first-hand how different academic disciplines fit together in addressing health problems. Using ethnography, I created an independent research project on the transmission of HIV among women in South America. In addition to performing interviews, I took photographs to document the project, which served as an important research tool and a creative outlet.

Again utilizing different angles in research, I completed a senior thesis evaluating the clinical use of art therapy in a community mental health setting. I particularly focused on the use of photography projects as a mental health empowerment tool in impoverished communities. The success of using an interdisciplinary approach to solve problems compelled me to explore health issues from a new perspective after graduation.

Interning at the Public Health Department after college, I designed and conducted a needs assessment on maternal depression in Latinas. The research I conducted in South America served as a conceptual foundation for the assessment. Although I found the work intellectually stimulating, I yearned for more interaction with patients and a deeper understanding of the biological underpinnings of illness.

Enrolling in a pre-medical post baccalaureate program, I thrived on the rigors of studying science in depth and found inspiration through international and local community work that enlivened the academic framework. Working in Central America on a summer medical mission to develop a cervical cancer prevention program, I performed breast exams, assisted with pap smears, and improved my Spanish as I educated patients about cervical cancer. Inspired by the few local doctors serving these communities, as they balanced their dual roles as clinicians and activists, I returned determined to reduce healthcare barriers in my own community. I immediately joined the local health clinic, where I counseled on preventative health and chronic diseases and took histories and vital signs. I found providing direct patient care immensely satisfying and realized that medicine involves the intellectual stimulation, emotional challenge, and chance to powerfully affect people's lives that I long for in a profession.

My current job, conducting psychosocial interviews for a study on HIV+ patients, has reinforced my passion for direct patient interaction while introducing me to a new medical perspective—end-of-life care. Working as a health coach, I witness how direct intervention can improve chronic care management in underserved populations. As I listen to patients in palliative care, I am cognizant of the crucial role compassionate medicine plays at the end of life and am reminded of the joy I feel when allowed to be present during intimate moments. It is in these moments with a patient near death that my heart begins beating a little faster—this time it is not with the joy of witnessing a new beginning but with comprehension of the end.

PERSONAL STATEMENT EXAMPLE 11
Foreign Applicant

I have noticed that many foreign applicants applying to US medical schools want to show how "American" they can be. I love the next personal statement because the author embraces her culture and uses it to make an excellent argument for combining Eastern and Western medical practices. If English is not your first language, be sure to have a native English speaker edit the essay for grammar.

I looked like a pin cushion with needles protruding from my face. The acupuncturist tweaked the needle inserted next to my eye to treat nearsightedness. My vision actually sharpened for a few days after the treatment. For scoliosis, I completely relaxed while a Chinese bone-setting doctor and her assistant pulled my arms and legs in opposite directions while I breathed out. My previously uneven shoulder blades have now flattened more evenly. The intriguing success of these healing techniques inspired my longstanding interest in complementary health improvement. At the age of twelve, I began Chinese acupuncture lessons and have since cultivated knowledge of culturally-sensitive medicine through international study, engaged in local clinical experiences, and performed lab research to explore the wonderful possibilities of healing.

Through studying abroad in India and Africa, I have immersed myself in cultural healing. As part of an international program, I initiated a trip to India to learn about Ayurveda/Siddha medicine. Far from its Chinese roots, I discovered patients who praised acupuncture's benefits for migraines. When I suggested combining acupuncture with the Indian herb *neem* known to relieve pain, the Indian patients' faces lit up at my interest in their traditional medicine. An extra open coconut to drink and a *bindi* on my forehead served as thanks. As an exchange student in Africa, I volunteered with the university's medical student-run clinic in black townships. White staff and black patients crowded in the mobile van with medical care bridging some of the gaping racial divide. I taught a little girl with fetal alcohol syndrome how to use a toothbrush and she threw some punches at me, an Asian who must know Kung Fu. We are from completely different worlds, but in the clinic we bonded over the goal of making her well. While in Africa, I also researched traditional healers. While I learned a great deal about culturally-sensitive medicine abroad, I further discovered the importance of engaging patients' cultural values to improve health close to home.

For three years, I worked as coordinator, intake leader, and Mandarin interpreter at a local free clinic serving a culturally-diverse, underprivileged population. In my multiple roles, I monitored patient flow, organized other undergraduates' shadowing opportunities, provided patients with referrals, and translated. I noted that I could optimally assist patients when I asked them about cultural attitudes towards health. I helped one Chinese patient by investigating how her Western medications might interact with the Chinese herbs she was taking. During a phone follow-up, she opened up to me about her desire to eat healthily and quit drinking. Through our shared cultural context, I suggested foods in the Chinese expression as less "hot" or greasy and more "cooling," such as drinking ginseng tea instead of alcohol. I started a ginseng regimen, and we shared various herbal recipes to maximize taste and effect. In a few months, she received her green card, and I coordinated my volunteer dates with her occasional visits to continue our culturally-appropriate dialogue.

My motivation to be an allopathic doctor stems from my frustration that I cannot pinpoint why acupuncture works or how an African shaman increases CD4 counts in AIDS patients. For two years, I have worked at a neuroscience lab, researching glucocorticoid mediation of learning, memory, and depression in mice while looking for behavior patterns. I hope my strong foundation in neuroscience will ultimately help me bridge the divide between traditional medicine and science by understanding the physiological basis for cultural medicine. But rather than working alone for hours in the dark mouse room, I wish to ponder the complexity of how lab science and cultural healing practices can be merged to improve health. Perhaps the combination of traditional healers dispensing foreign anti-retroviral medications will encourage an AIDS patient who has lost hope and resorted to reckless activity to practice safe behavior and take scientifically-tested medication.

As an allopathic doctor, I hope to combine my knowledge of Eastern and Western medicine. I want to find common grounds for traditional healing and behavioral responses based on scientific validation. I have witnessed how a handful of acupuncture needles and local anesthesia eliminate pain. One day I hope to understand what that needle near my eye did beneath the surface and be able to provide a scientifically justified hope for healing.

PERSONAL STATEMENT EXAMPLE 12
Military

This applicant dedicated her initial career to the military, where she creatively gained medical experience from both administrative and clinical angles. Though she will be leaving the army prior to attending medical school, she does an outstanding job of weaving her unique service experience into a story that demonstrates she possesses the qualities required to excel in medical school and beyond. Notice the strong hook whose theme runs through the entire essay and how each paragraph transitions seamlessly into the next.

*** Names have been changed to protect patient privacy

I will never forget them. Specialist (Spc.) Dvorak grasped my hand after being mortally wounded during a mortar attack in Basra, Iraq and a medical evacuation unit transported him to our facility. Though conscious upon arrival, he lost too much blood and passed away before my eyes while awaiting surgery. Muhammad Al-Jubouri drifted in and out of consciousness as the massive intracranial hemorrhage stole oxygen from his brain. He had been shot in combat while trying to harm American soldiers. "Stevo," the good-humored detainee, arched his back in agony as the tetanus infection he acquired after stepping on a nail in his compound spread to the muscles of his back. I felt helpless sitting and watching while these men suffered, always knowing I had the capability to do more. After leading in the US Army Medical Service Corps, witnessing family members struggle with life-threatening illness, and exploring multiple clinical experiences, I have confirmed my desire to become a physician who can use medical diplomacy and provide the best medical care for all in the United States and abroad.

Upon graduation from college, I entered the Medical Service Corps where I learned the diplomatic power of the medical profession and first became interested in the clinical side of medicine. Prior to deploying to Iraq, I was informed that the policy had shifted from winning hearts and minds because "it couldn't be done." However, during a fifteen-month deployment in the war zone, I witnessed the breakdown of cultural barriers through medical diplomacy on a daily basis. A detainee walking down the hall glaring at me with hatred, wanting to destroy me in an instant, might be in the hospital that night looking at me with vulnerability and hoping I could heal him. I took pride in our hospital providing exceptional care for all, despite political grumbles from back home complaining of US money being misspent on non-US citizens. My main military role involved serving in an administrative capacity and leading large staffs on all patient administration matters. I have saved lives through efficient patient evacuation, studied the financial aspects of the medical profession, and earned a military medal for creating a new detainee patient identification system. Though my formal administrative role provided critical support to the medical team, I always found myself wanting to delve more into the clinical arena and help patients like Spc. Dvorak, Muhammad Al-Jubouri, and Stevo.

I found myself gaining clinical experience in a way I never imagined. On October 21, 2006, my mom called to tell me my dad had been diagnosed with hepatitis C and she with stage 3 breast cancer one day later. I again felt helpless, but this time not hopeless. I watched as the clinical staff caring for my parents addressed not only their illness, but also their humanity. The staff playfully nicknamed my mom's wig, "Harriet," and joked with my dad about where he could find the same support in hepatitis C as my mom had in her "pink ribbon" fervor. Watching medicine from the patient side only increased my motivation to become a physician who can heal through a focus on treating the whole person.

After my parents regained their health with the help of an inspirational medical community, I devoted myself to finding out more about medicine from the provider side. Lunch breaks were soon filled with observing surgeries or autopsies. I creatively adapted my schedule to shadow an internist, obstetrician, and orthopedic surgeon. I soon found I would rather shadow a doctor on rounds than go home when my duty day ended. Eager to care for patients myself, I earned Emergency Medical Technician-Basic certification and thrived on using my skills to provide at least a small part of the healing process.

After years of military service and exploration of the medical field from both the patient and provider side, I strongly believe that amidst the political and ethical struggles, the beauty of serving others through medicine transcends cultural barriers and creates an even playing field for humanity. Doctors start a chain reaction by producing healthy individuals who can then contribute to society with their gifts and talents. I will never be able to go back and save Spc. Dvorak, Muhammad Al-Jubouri, and Stevo. However, I can change my role from supportive administrative staff to a leader on the team. I crave the knowledge that can change hearts and minds through medical diplomacy and look forward to providing the best possible medical care to all regardless of nationality, color, or creed.

PERSONAL STATEMENT EXAMPLE 13
Specialty Interest

This applicant already knows she wants to be an ophthalmologist. Though you certainly don't need to have your specialty chosen at this early stage, it is perfectly acceptable to mention a passion for a certain field if your life experiences establish a long-standing and consistent interest in a certain area. From the hook to the description of research, community service, and leadership activities, this applicant skillfully exhibits why she will be not only an excellent physician, but also an outstanding ophthalmologist.

"Hey, Four-Eyes! Watch out for the ball!" Before I could look up from my weathered copy of Charlotte's Web, a red dodge ball hit me square in the face. I looked down as shards of glass lay scattered on the ground – my guide to the outside world destroyed in an instant. I felt frustrated that I was the first student in Mrs. Morrison's third grade class to need glasses and often asked my parents why this was the case. They suggested I borrow books from the school library to learn more about the fascinating science of sight. Over time, I began to view my need for glasses as a blessing in disguise. This early experience introduced me to the thrill of discovering knowledge and ignited a passion for vision that has lasted long after the books were due. After exploring the world of eyesight as a bench researcher, community vision screener, overseas volunteer, and clinic founder, I am confident that serving as a physician will allow me to combine my dual passions for research and public health while drawing upon the skills gained from a sustained commitment to ophthalmology.

Pursuing multiple research opportunities in college allowed me to continue seeking answers to my own questions, while providing the freedom to think creatively and to test the limits of current scientific understanding. During my three years in an ophthalmology lab, we investigated the potential for gene therapy to treat blind patients who suffered from inherited retinal disease. As a recipient of the University Scholars Scholarship, I completed a senior thesis analyzing the precise anatomical changes in the retina of a mouse model for Leber's Congenital Amaurosis (LCA). The results of my study identified benchmark values that can be used when assessing the efficacy of new treatments for LCA in mouse models.

Outside of the laboratory, I wanted to learn how research findings could be practically applied to improve health outcomes. I volunteered with a non-profit dedicated to improving sight for underprivileged communities and provided preliminary vision screenings at local health fairs. As community advocates, we relied on evidence-based interventions to engage and educate individuals who lacked access to vision services. Furthermore, we referred these individuals to other free national eye-coverage programs, thereby ensuring their continued vision care.

I then sought to gain a greater understanding of global health concerns by volunteering with the same non-profit in India. In a dusty village 20 miles from the state capital, a large crowd of men, women, children, goats, and cows stared back at us with mutual fascination. We screened hundreds of people for vision problems ranging from childhood refractive errors to adult macular degeneration. I noticed Swapna, whose warm mahogany skin glowed in stark contrast to her icy blue eyes. I soon realized her blue eyes stemmed not from genetics, but from cataracts that resulted in near-blindness. We took Swapna back to the capital, and the next day, she received cataract surgery. Within minutes, the ophthalmologist had replaced her opaque lens with a new artificial one. A few days later, Swapna's grandson clung to her paisley sari as a doctor removed the eye patch. While I could not understand the native tongue, I could feel Swapna's happiness as she conversed with the grandchild to whom she had often spoken, yet had never seen. She smiled while touching the boy's eyes, nose, and mouth, as if trying to translate his face into a new language. I was moved by the ophthalmologist's use of simple yet sophisticated methods to radically improve an individual's quality of life.

Inspired by my India experience, I felt compelled to act after learning of Sri Lanka's alarmingly high prevalence of untreated diabetic retinopathy. I proposed a clinic model that would provide a complete screening for diabetic retinopathy at no cost to the patient. I relished the challenge to incorporate international standards of care while ensuring the program remained relevant to Sri Lanka's unique cultural context. I became acutely aware of the complexities of modern healthcare delivery as we delicately balanced the desire to provide the best quality of care with real-world constraints, such as rising medical costs and patient compliance. Undeterred by physicians' initial hesitation to work with someone so young, I successfully harnessed the skills and talents of numerous physicians in order to create an efficient method of screening and caring for diabetic patients and their families.

Each of my clinical experiences has demonstrated the importance of timely public health interventions to improving the health of populations. As these experiences have been largely independent ventures based on my own initiative, I will adopt a more structured approach to furthering my understanding of health policies and practices by enrolling in the Master's of Public Health program in England this fall. Upon completing the MPH, I look forward to entering medical school and continuing my pursuit of a medical career dedicated to making a tangible impact on the lives of individual patients and underserved communities in the United States and abroad.

PERSONAL STATEMENT EXAMPLE 14
Relationships

Building relationships is a large part of doctoring. This applicant wisely recognizes the importance of personal communication and relationship building in her life and desire to become a physician. Look how she uses the metaphor of being invited to frame an intriguing essay focused on relationships.

It was 5:30 am, Ghanaian time. I would normally have been reluctant to wake up at such an early hour but had not been able to sleep much with baby Wisdom suffering from malaria and needing close observation. Feet pattered on the rough concrete floor as children wandered into hallways sleepily brushing their teeth. A voice called out for Ema, Polly, Christopher, and Ernestine to receive the HIV medication that had to be taken at 6:00 am, every morning, most likely for the rest of their lives. It was a day like any other of the 14 days I spent volunteering in a Ghanaian orphanage. As I helped serve each orphan their daily breakfast of rice porridge, one of the children solemnly said to me, as Ghanaians traditionally do before eating a meal, "You are invited." Those words have resonated with me since. I felt deeply honored to be invited into each of these children's lives and this feeling of privilege drives me towards a career in medicine. Through raising funds to build primary schools in Uganda, researching Alzheimer's disease, and interning at a children's hospital, I am consistently driven by the importance of relationships in improving lives.

My involvement in student-run undergraduate activities has shown me the power of using relationships to improve the lives of those in need. I joined a non-profit focused on building schools because of its capacity to permanently change the lives of Ugandan children with no school to attend. As an executive board member for the next two years, I saw firsthand that strengthening relationships between members solidified the effort to impact change and bring about results. I therefore devoted my leadership to ensuring each member felt welcomed to the group and to acknowledging their efforts. We raised over $20,000 to build primary schools in Uganda.

Fascinated by the power of relationships, I sought to research Alzheimer's disease, an illness that tragically takes away the power of knowing another person. My grandfather was diagnosed with the neurodegenerative disorder when I was young, and I saw the devastating effects it had on his relationships with friends and family. Through trial and error in the lab, I learned to ask for help when unsure about a step in the procedure and how working as a unified team brought about the best results. The research also reiterated the importance of careful attention to detail.

Yearning for more direct patient contact, I experienced firsthand the reward of developing a meaningful connection with a patient during my internship at a children's hospital. My first day on the pediatric floor, I entered a room to find Shavasia, a 6-year-old girl undergoing chemotherapy treatments, lying in bed screaming in discomfort while her mother tried desperately to calm her. Slightly alarmed but undeterred, I told Shavasia about all of the crafts we would do in the playroom, the games we would play, and the other children she would meet. By pointing out toys and games she might be interested in at the playroom, I tried my best to make Shavasia feel at ease. Soon playing happily with other patients, she said to her mother, "This is so fun I forgot we were in a hospital!" That offhand comment and the gratitude on her mother's face gave me a sense of fulfillment I hope to attain everyday. Through my efforts, I helped Shavasia feel more comfortable despite the circumstances that brought her to the hospital. She has returned for more treatments and, each time, I make sure to visit Shavasia and ask how she is doing. It is these kinds of long-term relationships and other meaningful experiences in the lives of others that drive me towards becoming a physician.

Each encounter with somebody who needs my help, whether it is to hold a mother's child while she gets tested for HIV in Ghana, to work with others in researching a devastating disease, or to explain procedures to young patients in ways they can understand, is akin to being invited to take a look into a tiny part of their lives. Once that window is opened, there is an invaluable opportunity to improve that person's life in some way and to leave a lasting impression. It is the doctor's privilege to be connected to another person in such an intimate way. I strive to become a doctor who patients feel comfortable with – to become a doctor whose patients will, just like the children I met in Ghana, want to invite me into their lives.

Appendix II
AMCAS and TMDSAS Work/Activities Examples

Nontraditional applicants that took time off between college and medical school wrote most of the following examples and created outstanding AMCAS work/activities essays without filling up every slot. The third example shows the quality required of every activity if you are going to include 15 experiences. Given the TMDSAS work/activities section is slightly different than the AMCAS, the final example includes both AMCAS and TMDSAS entries from the same applicant for you to see how the same information is modified to meet the requirements of each application type. To maintain privacy, I removed or changed all personal information including contact name and title, organization name, and city/state/country. Don't forget this information will be required when you fill out the AMCAS or TMDSAS work/activities sections.

AMCAS WORK/ACTIVITIES EXAMPLE 1

This applicant pursued other careers for over twenty years before applying to medical school. Though he could have included hundreds of interesting work/activities in the AMCAS application, he adeptly included only his eight strongest experiences. He avoided the common mistake of bogging the application down in superfluous details and consciously focuses the admissions committee on his most impressive life achievements.

Experience Type: Community Service/Volunteer – Medical/Clinical
Most Meaningful Experience: Yes
Experience Name: HIV Counselor/Clinic Assistant
Dates: 06/2010 – Present
Total Hours: 999
Experience Description: Motivated by caring for friends dying of AIDS in the 1990s, I have become a certified HIV counselor providing pre- and post-test HIV counseling to a high-risk population at a community-based clinic. I conduct individual counseling sessions that include risk assessment, discussion of harm reduction goals, motivational interviewing, preparation of harm-reduction plans, and referrals to primary care, mental health, and substance abuse services. I administer HIV tests and give test results, both positive and negative.

Most Meaningful Experience Remarks: During this counseling experience, I have been challenged by difficult discussions with individuals who want to contract HIV, adults afraid of any sexual contact for fear of infection, minors engaging in unprotected sex with adults, and clients afraid to tell partners of their status. In addition to active counseling, I participate in regular continuing education activities. I also perform STD testing for symptomatic and asymptomatic clients, run routine laboratory tests, and administer STD treatment. Working one-on-one with individuals struggling with the effects of a chronic disease confirmed my desire to enter medicine and focus on caring for others through primary care.

Experience Type: Community Service/Volunteer – Medical/Clinical
Most Meaningful Experience: Yes
Experience Name: Designer/Programmer: Electronic Medical Record and Case Management System/Clinic Assistant
Dates: 05/2010 – 04/2013
Total Hours: 999
Dates: 05/2013 – Present
Total Hours: 650
Experience Description: I volunteered at an acute care clinic and community center that acts as a "point of entry" and health care system guide to a mostly immigrant population. As a clinic assistant, I took patients' vital signs, ran

routine laboratory tests, performed immunizations and PPDs, filled prescriptions, and processed referrals to primary care, social service, and mental health providers. Seeing an opportunity to use my programming skills to benefit the clinic, I now serve as one of two principal developers of a web-based medical record and case management system.

Most Meaningful Experience Remarks: Volunteering at the clinic provided a window into the difficult medical problems faced by immigrants and disadvantaged populations and allowed me to follow patients with various diseases including diabetes, COPD, work-related fractures, severe skin infections, depression, and high blood pressure. In addition to my hands on work in the clinic, I used my computer skills to develop a system that provides case management functions, electronic medical records using a SOAP format, prevention information, and accurate demographic data to serve as the basis for grant writing. Because the clinic operates at different sites across the county, the system is designed to be easily accessed anywhere while maintaining client confidentiality.

Experience Type: Teaching/Tutoring/Teaching Assistant
Most Meaningful Experience: No
Experience Name: Teaching Assistant, General Chemistry
Dates: 08/2010 – 05/2011
Total Hours: 400
Experience Description: As a general chemistry teaching assistant, I prepared and taught a weekly general chemistry workshop to undergraduate and post-baccalaureate pre-medical students. I separately tutored small groups and individuals selected by the instructor as requiring the most assistance. Because many students doubted their abilities and often feared the material, I helped them build confidence and analytical skills through successful problem solving. I also ran popular comprehensive midterm and final review sessions.

Experience Type: Teaching/Tutoring/Teaching Assistant
Most Meaningful Experience: No
Experience Name: Private Tutor, General Physics
Dates: 05/2010 – 10/2011
Total Hours: 250

Experience Description: After serving as a chemistry teaching assistant, several of my post-baccalaureate students asked me to privately tutor them in physics. I prepared practice exercises for our weekly meetings and carefully structured the problem-solving exercises to match each student's current grasp of the material. It was quite satisfying to witness each student improve in both skill and confidence through the semester, with one student increasing her C grade to an A.

Experience Type: Research/Lab
Most Meaningful Experience: No
Experience Name: Research Assistant
Dates: 10/2012 – 12/2013
Total Hours: 600
Experience Description: I worked at a laboratory studying the social function of emotions. As a research assistant, I coordinated data collection to examine shifts in self-understanding during experiences of compassion and pride. I collected EKG and skin conductance data from subjects exposed to emotionally-powerful stimuli. I then wrote a program to rapidly aggregate physiological data, greatly improving the efficiency of a process formerly done by hand and allowing a more complete profile of subjects' emotional reactivity.

Experience Type: Research/Lab
Most Meaningful Experience: Yes
Experience Name: Research Assistant
Dates: 10/2007 – 12/2008
Total Hours: 999
Experience Description: I joined this psychology laboratory to further my interest in the social function and physiological basis of emotions. I started on a project examining the emotional functioning of patients with Alzheimer's disease and frontotemporal lobar degeneration (FTLD), and then became lead research assistant on a study of linguistic patterns in patients with dementia. I was also part of a team analyzing heterosexual, lesbian, and gay couples' communication patterns and physiological responses during stressful conversations. While working in the lab, I participated in weekly lab meetings and literature reviews.

Most Meaningful Experience Remarks: This was my first substantial clinical research experience and provided an excellent introduction into the interaction between emotions and health. While studying the emotional functioning of patients with Alzheimer's disease and FTLD, I helped guide subjects through a series of emotion-inducing tasks (such as recalling their wedding day) while recording their physiological reactions, facial expressions, and subjective experience. After six months in the lab, I received a promotion to lead research assistant on a study of linguistic patterns in patients with dementia. We measured the degree to which patients' language reflected a connection to bodily and emotional experience, looking for linguistic patterns that might provide subtle signs of dementia onset and possibly serve as the basis for an inexpensive screening tool. During this project, I coordinated the activities of other research assistants and wrote computer programs to help analyze patients' memories of significant events (like JFK's assassination). I enjoyed every aspect of clinical research, from the individual interaction with each research subject to analyzing the data to manuscript creation.

Experience Type: Paid Employment – Not Medical/Clinical
Most Meaningful Experience: No
Experience Name: Computer Programmer and Systems Analyst
Dates: 02/2006 – 01/2007
Total Hours: 999
Dates: 02/2007 – 01/2008
Total Hours: 999
Dates: 02/2008 – 01/2009
Total Hours: 999
Dates: 02/2009 – Present
Total Hours: 999
Experience Description: While finishing my undergraduate degree and taking premedical courses, I have worked as a systems analyst and computer programmer in the information technology department of a nationally known 350-person law firm. I write programs to analyze business workflows, such as expense reimbursement. The job requires frequent interaction with and technical education of various constituencies including partners, junior attorneys, technical staff, secretaries, and software vendors. While in school, I was asked

to serve as interim manager of a firm-wide upgrade to the desktop operating and document management systems. I write programs in C#, Java, JavaScript and VB.NET.

Experience Type: Community Service/Volunteer – Medical/Clinical
Most Meaningful Experience: No
Experience Name: Preparing and Serving Food to People in Need
Dates: 01/2012 – Present
Total Hours: 500
Experience Description: I help prepare, cook, and serve weekly meals at a "free restaurant" providing a hot meal to anyone who comes through the doors. I enjoy the simple work of preparing meals because of the great respect offered to those who arrived to receive food. The atmosphere cultivated is not that of the more fortunate helping the less fortunate, but rather that of fellow human beings helping each other. My appreciation for this ethos has led me to seek out other organizations grounded in the ideal of a community caring for its own members.

AMCAS WORK/ACTIVITIES EXAMPLE 2

This applicant had over 20 possible experiences to include but successfully picked the top 14. It was difficult for her to select three most meaningful activities, but she wisely chose experiences where she exhibited commitment and leadership, two of the most important qualities admissions committees look for in applicants.

Experience Type: Community Service/Volunteer – Medical/Clinical
Most Meaningful Experience: No
Experience Name: Trainer for Emergency Department Volunteers
Dates: 01/2011 – Present
Total Hours: 500
Experience Description: After almost one year of volunteering, I was chosen to be a new volunteer trainer. New volunteers must undergo a rigorous five-hour "secondary" training before they are granted a shift of their own. I train approximately one person a week, focusing on teaching how to advocate for patients, assist with traumas, follow universal precautions, deliver lab speci-

mens, and fetch supplies. I also train new volunteers to appropriately answer patient questions, preserve patient privacy, and safely assist with procedures.

Experience Type: Community Service/Volunteer – Medical/Clinical
Most Meaningful Experience: Yes
Experience Name: Clinic Volunteer
Dates: 09/2010 – Present
Total Hours: 800
Experience Description: The clinic serves the long-term health needs of the low-income community surrounding the general hospital. More than half of our patients are uninsured with the majority being treated for substance abuse. Many don't speak English or are former prison inmates, and many have been coming to the clinic all their lives. My tasks involve taking patient vital signs, interviewing patients, charting histories, writing orders, and preparing patients for lab tests. I maintain an efficient flow in the clinic by rooming patients, notifying doctors of waiting patients, and quickly cleaning rooms as doctors complete each exam.
Most Meaningful Experience Remarks: Working at the clinic serving a mostly uninsured and disadvantaged population provided a contrast to my experience volunteering in the emergency department. In the clinic, I enjoyed developing long-term relationships with patients who often felt helpless and left out of society. I thoroughly enjoyed one-on-one contact with the patients and learning the art of taking a history and ordering tests based on a differential diagnosis. Beyond my usual clinic responsibilities, I assisted the head nurse with other tasks such as preparing for visits from the mammogram van, coordinating with the hospital to repair the EKG machine, and running nutrition classes for diabetic patients.

Experience Type: Community Service/Volunteer – Medical/Clinical
Most Meaningful Experience: No
Experience Name: Caseworker
Dates: 06/2010 – Present
Total Hours: 600
Experience Description: The clinic provides myriad services to the homeless including medical, psychological, dental, optometric, legal, foot washing, and clothing donation. I record clients' social histories and accompany them

throughout their clinic visits, ensuring they receive the appropriate services. While serving as a foot-washer at the women's clinic, I researched and implemented improved disinfecting procedures for the foot washing basins. I have also shadowed a clinic doctor, medical student, and caseworkers to further observe health education in a free-clinic setting.

Experience Type: Community Service/Volunteer – Medical/Clinical
Most Meaningful Experience: Yes
Experience Name: Emergency Department Volunteer
Dates: 03/2010 – Present
Total Hours: 999
Experience Description: In this role, patient advocacy is my first priority. I perform tasks that doctors and staff are often too busy to do: reassuring patients and family members, bringing patients food, water, and warm blankets, and looking for lost belongings. I also assist doctors and nurses with traumas by fetching equipment, performing CPR, and helping with non-invasive procedures.

Most Meaningful Experience Remarks: Volunteering in a level I trauma center that mainly serves the underprivileged, I have assisted a wide variety of patients including those with life-threatening medical conditions, surgical patients, and victims of violent crimes. Spending a significant time in the emergency department allowed me to witness the demands on physicians and the stresses on patients who are suffering. I have learned to communicate with those who are unable to speak, currently incarcerated, mentally unstable, and under the influence of drugs. I have also assisted with the after-death care and transport of patients who have passed away. After about a year of volunteering, I was chosen to be a new volunteer trainer responsible for preparing future volunteers.

Experience Type: Conferences Attended
Most Meaningful Experience: No
Experience Name: Practicing Medicine/Providing Healthcare
Dates: 08/2010 – 08/2010
Total Hours: 40
Experience Description: "Practicing Medicine/Providing Healthcare" was a weeklong conference for individuals seriously considering a career in medi-

cine. In the mornings, I attended lectures on a variety of topics including the economics, politics, and daily life of various types of doctors and researchers. In the afternoons, I participated in hospital rounds and doctor shadowing in the general medicine, cardiac catheterization, pediatric outpatient, and primary care internal medicine departments.

Experience Type: Teaching/Tutoring/Teaching Assistant
Most Meaningful Experience: No
Experience Name: Teaching Assistant, General Chemistry
Dates: 08/2009 – 05/2010
Total Hours: 400
Experience Description: As a teaching assistant in general chemistry, I taught a weekly workshop to a group of undergraduate and post-baccalaureate students. I tutored several students individually and in pairs, assisting them with homework and exam preparation. The professor chose students in need of the most assistance. However, as other students expressed interest in my help, I made time to tutor an additional student outside of the official duties. I also taught periodic exam review sessions to large groups of students and graded laboratory reports.

Experience Type: Paid Employment – Medical/Clinical
Most Meaningful Experience: No
Experience Name: Telemedical Research and Development Intern
Dates: 06/2009 – 08/2009
Total Hours: 300
Experience Description: In areas lacking specialists, primary care physicians can request a specialist consultation using "store-and-forward" telemedicine applications. These applications transmit patient information and digital images to the specialist for review. At a company that makes telemedicine hardware and software, I performed extensive medical literature research to understand what information ophthalmologists and infectious disease specialists require to make remote diagnoses. I gained a high-level understanding of the main ophthalmologic disorders and infectious diseases, determined which were possible to diagnose remotely, and used existing paper consultation forms to design web-based forms.

Experience Type: Conferences Attended
Most Meaningful Experience: No
Experience Name: Mini Medical School
Dates: 04/2007 – 06/2007
Total Hours: 18
Dates: 04/2008 – 06/2008
Total Hours: 18
Dates: 04/2010 – 06/2010
Total Hours: 18
Experience Description: I attended this six-week lecture series in the spring of 2007, 2008, and 2010. I have learned about subjects ranging from fetal surgery to pain management. On the "Elective Saturdays," I frequented the anatomy lab and enjoyed handling the dissections. In the health research sections, I learned how to research medical information on the Web, which later proved useful in my job as a telemedical research and development intern.

Experience Type: Paid Employment – Not Medical/Clinical
Most Meaningful Experience: Yes
Experience Name: Software Developer, Manager, and Manager of Multiple Teams
Dates: 10/1995 – 09/1999
Total Hours: 999
Dates: 10/2000 – 03/2004
Total Hours: 999
Experience Description: I spent nine years working full time (40 hours/week) in the software field. My company is known for databases that store massive quantities of information in a secure and organized way and applications for businesses to access that information. From 1995-1999, I developed and maintained the software installation programs for all products. From 2000 through 2003, I managed two teams to perform the duties I had previously been doing myself. From 2003 through 2004, I managed my teams' transition to a new organization, where we designed and developed a Java-based Contact Management application, as well as instituted new internal development and release processes.
Most Meaningful Experience Remarks: Working as a software developer and manager honed my analytical, leadership, and teamwork skills. Collaborating

with multiple organizations, I created the company's first installable patch pro-cedure, trial product release, and Windows CD. Then, to meet the needs of this fast-paced company, I managed a team that reduced the trial release process from eight weeks to one week and completely re-designed the database instal-lation to work on both Windows and UNIX platforms. During my time at the company, I worked my way up from software developer to manager to manager of multiple teams, while also being given the task to manage a quality assurance team located in India. I thrived in the fast-pace environment of the software world but longed for a way to make a more direct impact on the health of indi-viduals. I look forward to bringing my problem-solving, communication, and leadership skills to medicine.

Experience Type: Paid Employment – Not Medical/Clinical
Most Meaningful Experience: No
Experience Name: Director of Program Management
Dates: 03/2004 – 08/2008
Total Hours: 999
Dates: 09/2008 – 05/2011
Total Hours: 999
Dates: 06/2011 – Present
Total Hours: 999
Experience Description: While I am now part-time, I worked at a Silicon Valley software firm full-time from 2004 through 2008. As Director of Program Management, I managed the logistical, tactical, and scheduling aspects of all product releases. While attending a post-baccalaureate program full-time from 2008-2011, I worked for the firm part-time and managed the implementa-tion of an automated process for digitally signing product releases. From June 2011-present, I have worked part-time as the technical liaison to a leading soft-ware company to resolve issues with their software, communicate information about upcoming product releases, and drive the adoption of appropriate new technologies.

Experience Type: Community Service/Volunteer – Medical/Clinical
Most Meaningful Experience: No
Experience Name: Emergency Response Team Leader

Dates: 10/1995 – 03/2004
Total Hours: 500
Experience Description: As Team Leader for a volunteer organization serving the Silicon Valley firm's campus, I received training in First Aid, CPR, and evacuation procedures. I helped evacuate the headquarters' buildings during alarms and bomb threats, both practice and real. I wrote extensive safety literature and distributed it to my department and the rest of the Emergency Response Team.

Experience Type: Other
Most Meaningful Experience: No
Experience Name: Deaf Community Experiences
Dates: 08/1993 – 06/1994
Total Hours: 100
Experience Description: My introduction to Deaf culture began in college when I joined the American Sign Language (ASL) club and was admitted to the first ASL class offered there. The late Marie Jean Philip, a prominent and groundbreaking figure in the Deaf community, taught the class. As part of my coursework, I attended Deaf cultural events, such as plays, parties, and poetry readings, and conversed in ASL with the people I met. Doctors who can communicate with the Deaf are in short supply, and I hope to join forces with other doctors in assisting this community.

Experience Type: Artistic Endeavors
Most Meaningful Experience: No
Experience Name: Singer and Musician
Dates: 09/2001 – 08/2006
Total Hours: 999
Dates: 09/2006 – 08/2011
Total Hours: 999
Dates: 09/2011 – Present
Total Hours: 700
Experience Description: As a child, I learned ukulele and took piano and harp lessons. In college, I joined my university a cappella singing group and became well known for my ability to imitate a trumpet using only my mouth.

I created the group's first intersession tour by marketing our services to northeastern businesses. After college I joined an award-winning, four-woman a cappella group and sang with them for eight years. I have also performed with many other groups and am a session singer at a local record label, often writing backup, lead, and instrumental vocal parts on the spot for a large number of musical groups and film productions.

AMCAS WORK/ACTIVITIES EXAMPLE 3

A rare applicant who had enough spectacular experiences to fill all 15 allotted spaces wrote the example below. If you are wavering on whether or not to include an experience in your application, look to this example to see the quality required. Remember, don't fill the space just to fill the space. The admissions committees can see through "fluffy" activities. Please note identifying data has been removed from all of these AMCAS work/activities models. When writing your AMCAS, be sure to be specific and use proper names, as opposed to the generic names provided in these examples.

Experience Type: Paid Employment – Medical/Clinical
Most Meaningful Experience: No
Experience Name: Clinical Research Coordinator
Dates: 10/2013 – Present
Total Hours: 999
Experience Description: Motivated by a desire to gain greater clinical exposure, I currently work as a clinical research coordinator for a study examining the safety and effectiveness of a device used during glaucoma filtration surgery (trabeculectomy). I liaise between the sponsor and all eight sites and communicate daily with physicians, research coordinators, and regulatory personnel. Coordinating all data collection and analysis requires strong communication and problem-solving skills. I have improved my ability to multi-task and manage competing demands between our site and other study sites. I enjoy interacting with patients, shadowing ophthalmologists weekly, and observing surgeries.

Experience Type: Honors/Awards/Recognitions
Most Meaningful Experience: No

Experience Name: Awards and Honors
Dates: 09/2012 – 05/2013
Total Hours: 0
Experience Description: In recognition of my academic and extra-curricular achievements during my university career, I was named a finalist for the Rhodes Scholarship in September 2012. I was also placed on the Dean's List for the 2011-2012 academic year for achieving a GPA above a 3.7 and received a Bachelor's of Arts in Biology magna cum laude for maintaining a cumulative GPA above 3.6 during my undergraduate career.

Experience Type: Honors/Awards/Recognitions
Most Meaningful Experience: No
Experience Name: Top 10 College Women
Dates: 09/2012
Total Hours: 0
Experience Description: A leading US magazine named me one of the "Top 10 College Women." I was selected from college seniors across the US and Canada for this award valued at $5,000. Selection was based upon academic achievement, leadership experience, and involvement in community and campus affairs. Additionally, I was the recipient of the Beauty of Giving Award, chosen from among the "Top 10 College Women" award winners for a $3,000 cash prize based on outstanding community service work.

Experience Type: Paid Employment – Medical/Clinical
Most Meaningful Experience: No
Experience Name: Research Intern
Dates: 05/2012 – 7/2012
Total Hours: 500
Experience Description: I interned in the Health System Planning and Research Branch to understand how governmental health policies are informed and implemented. I worked on the "Externally-Informed Annual Health Systems Trends Report" exploring challenges to public health systems, both in Canada and abroad. I performed a literature search on health services research and identified relevant primary literature. Based on my performance, I wrote the section entitled, "Chronic Disease Prevention and Management," which

critically evaluated more than 70 research articles. Overall, I became aware of the complexity of health care systems and the political, economic, and social contexts in which medicine is practiced.

Experience Type: Honors/Awards/Recognitions
Most Meaningful Experience: No
Experience Name: Named a "Young Leader of Social Change"
Dates: 04/2012 – 4/2013
Total Hours: 0
Experience Description: I received this award in both 2012 and 2013. I was recognized for my work helping to improve vision both locally and internationally, as well as for my independent projects with the Clinic for Diabetic Retinopathy (2012) and for my research project in Bangladesh (2013). As a result, I was asked to speak at a global health innovation summit in 2012 and 2013.

Experience Type: Community Service/Volunteer – Medical/Clinical
Most Meaningful Experience: No
Experience Name: Peer Advisor
Dates: 09/2011 – 05/2013
Total Hours: 100
Experience Description: I worked in conjunction with faculty, academic advisors, and house deans to help incoming freshmen transition to college life. I aided students in class selection and addressed non-academic concerns that arose during the summer before college. I enjoyed participating in New Student Orientation for incoming freshmen and remaining in contact with students throughout the academic year. As an advisor specifically for other University Scholars, I also helped students contact potential mentors for their independent research. I am confident my ability to work collaboratively with numerous faculty members has prepared me well for a career in medicine that necessitates teamwork and cooperation.

Experience Type: Research/Lab
Most Meaningful Experience: Yes
Experience Name: Independent Research Project
Dates: 08/2011 – 8/2012

Total Hours: 300

Experience Description: To augment my extracurricular work aimed at addressing avoidable blindness, I conducted research on childhood blindness in Bangladesh. I had read a paper reporting that girls in Bangladesh were significantly more likely than boys to suffer from preventable blindness. However, no reasons were provided for this finding. Thus, I proposed a research project to further examine the factors that put Bangladeshi girls at a greater risk of becoming blind due to preventable causes than boys. To answer this question, I surveyed the primary caregivers of 88 blind children and 264 non-blind children in a case-controlled epidemiological study.

Most Meaningful Experience Remarks: This experience was meaningful because it allowed me to apply all of my skills and knowledge gained from biology, sociology, and statistics courses to a topic I was passionate about. In addition to proposing, organizing, and obtaining IRB approval for the study, I created a novel 50-item questionnaire to obtain information about family structure, education level, socio-economic status, and health beliefs, attitudes, and practices. I also conducted several field tests of the survey to ensure the questions were culturally sensitive while remaining clinically relevant. Overall, I found the factors most predictive of childhood blindness in girls included mother's educational status, mother's comfort with seeking medical attention for her child, and the child's nutritional status. Although I worked under the guidance of professors from the US and England, neither was present during the data collection stage. As a result, the project required independence and self-directed learning. Living and working in the same villages as the subjects I interviewed also required me to be versatile and adaptable, as I had to overcome any unexpected challenges on my own in an unfamiliar setting.

Experience Type: Leadership - Not Listed Elsewhere
Most Meaningful Experience: Yes
Experience Name: Founder
Dates: 09/2010 – Present
Total Hours: 999

Experience Description: In the summer of 2010, I read the prevalence of diabetes in Sri Lanka was approximately ten times the global level. At the time, only one clinic in the capital city of Colombo was capable of carrying out the tests needed for a comprehensive diagnosis of diabetic retinopathy, a common complication of diabetes. Yet, the cost of the tests was prohibitively expensive for the average Sri Lankan. Over the course of the next year, I performed research to draft a proposal for a clinic that would provide free vision screenings and follow-up for diabetic retinopathy according to standards set forth by the World Health Organization's Vision 2020 Initiative.

Most Meaningful Experience Remarks: My involvement was meaningful as it represented a sustained commitment to helping solve a problem that others had previously recognized but never acted on. I spent several months in Sri Lanka between 2010 and 2011 to help establish the clinic and have traveled back to visit the clinic every few months. I gained a solid understanding of the state of vision care in Sri Lanka, and then designed a proposal for the clinic based on what I had observed as strengths and weaknesses of the current system. Through this project, I became familiar with medical terminology relating to this area of medicine as I read textbooks and clinical guidelines to understand international standards for care of diabetic retinopathy. This experience demanded professionalism and strong communication skills as I collaborated with physicians, hospital administrators, representatives from the Sri Lankan Ministry of Healthcare and Nutrition, and potential funding partners. I persistently presented my plan for the clinic both confidently and knowledgeably to articulate why exactly this model, proposed by a young student raised abroad, provided a novel method for addressing a growing problem in Sri Lanka. The clinic now screens and provides follow-up care for hundreds of patients each month.

Experience Type: Research/Lab
Most Meaningful Experience: Yes
Experience Name: Research Assistant
Dates: 09/2010 – 9/2013
Total Hours: 999
Experience Description: I helped design research protocols and tested animal subjects to explore the potential for gene therapy in patients with inherited eye diseases causing severe visual impairment and blindness. I worked alongside other lab members on projects utilizing techniques such as cryosectioning, microscopy, retinal dissection, perfusion, and testing of the optokinetic

nystagmus reflex (OKR). This early commitment to the lab gave me the background and confidence needed to pose my own scientific questions. For my senior thesis, I wanted to find out how the retinal anatomy of the CEP290 -/- mouse (a model for Leber's Congenital Amaurosis in humans) changes during the postnatal weeks 1-6.

Most Meaningful Experience Remarks: This experience was meaningful because it allowed me to gain a deeper understanding of the process of translational research. I used microscopy, pupillometry, and a test of the OKR to find that CEP290 -/- mice are born with photoreceptor cells, but these cells degenerate with time and cause the retina to thin. The inner and outer segments, the outer nuclear layer, and the outer plexiform layer are particularly vulnerable to degeneration. This data can then be used as a baseline against which to measure the effectiveness of proposed gene therapy treatments. Working in basic research challenged me to be diligent, patient, and persistent. Additionally, the lab introduced me to the potential end results of successful translational research. The principal investigator was treating LCA in 12 individuals in a clinical trial using AAV injection, and I helped analyze the study data. It was extremely rewarding to observe the patients' marked improvement in vision and quality of life following the treatment. This remarkable experience has inspired me to remain committed to translational research throughout my future career in medicine.

Experience Type: Research/Lab
Most Meaningful Experience: No
Experience Name: Research Assistant
Dates: 09/2010 – 8/2012
Total Hours: 400
Experience Description: Over the course of two years, I became familiar with all stages of research study design, implementation, and reporting. I worked on a study examining the influence of nurse staffing on patient outcomes in the Neonatal Intensive Care Unit. I helped recruit hospitals, amend the survey, and manage a database of 104 hospitals and more than 5,000 nurses. I also used statistical packages such as SPSS to make regression models and other data analyses. I prepared initial drafts of manuscripts and assisted in writing NIH grants for the center. The experience reinforced the need for collaboration and

teamwork in patient care and the invaluable role of nurses in improving patient outcomes.

Experience Type: Community Service/Volunteer – Medical/Clinical
Most Meaningful Experience: No
Experience Name: Global Impact Corps Volunteer
Dates: 06/2010 – 07/2010
Total Hours: 240
Experience Description: I worked alongside ophthalmologists, optometrists, and other volunteers based at an eye clinic in Chennai, India. I learned how to test a patient's visual acuity and use a slit lamp. We traveled to villages, slums, and schools to provide free vision screenings to low-income individuals. I observed cataract surgeries and regularly shadowed the doctors. Additionally, I participated in outreach programs to teach individuals about good health practices needed to protect one's vision. From this hands-on experience, I gained appreciation for an integrated approach to patient care, which incorporates research evidence, public health initiatives, and direct patient care.

Experience Type: Extracurricular Activities
Most Meaningful Experience: No
Experience Name: Pilates
Dates: 09/2009 – Present
Total Hours: 300
Experience Description: During my college career, I enjoyed participating in Pilates group classes as a way of unwinding in a healthy and productive manner. I took reformer and matte Pilates classes at my university and a private studio. Pilates is based on precise, controlled movements that require steady concentration. I found it rewarding to see the gradual changes in my body that resulted from consistent dedication to the Pilates methods. I eventually sought to introduce others to my love of Pilates and completed training to become a Pilates Method Alliance-certified Beginner Matte instructor in October 2012.

Experience Type: Community Service/Volunteer – Medical/Clinical
Most Meaningful Experience: No
Experience Name: Board Member

Dates: 09/2009 – 05/2013

Total Hours: 300

Experience Description: I served as a volunteer with my university's chapter of a community organization dedicated to helping improving the vision of all for four years. As the chair of vision screenings, I organized and conducted vision screenings at soup kitchens and schools in the inner city. I also assisted with leading community health fairs that provided education on eye health and referrals to free vision care. Additionally, as vice president, I helped the chapter secure increased funding from the university. I was named Chapter Volunteer of the Year in 2010 when I helped raise over $1,500 for international programs.

Experience Type: Teaching/Tutoring/Teaching Assistant

Most Meaningful Experience: No

Experience Name: Elementary School Tutor

Dates: 09/2009 – 5/2010

Total Hours: 80

Experience Description: I volunteered at an elementary school in the inner city. Each week, I tutored and mentored second grade students performing below grade level in math and English. I honed my communication skills as I catered to each student's needs and creatively devised reinforcement activities drawing upon the student's personal interests to make the coursework more relevant. I also completed cultural sensitivity training to gain a better understanding of the diverse demographic and socioeconomic traits of the students. I enjoyed being able to tangibly measure the students' progress during the course of the year through improved test scores and reading abilities.

Experience Type: Honors/Awards/Recognitions

Most Meaningful Experience: No

Experience Name: University Scholars Scholarship

Dates: 09/2009

Total Hours: 0

Experience Description: I was one of twenty-five freshmen students from an incoming class of over 2,500 awarded this research scholarship. I was selected based on my research pursuits in high school and my expressed interest in pursuing independent research projects in university. The scholarship included funding for all research activities (I secured a $3,000 grant to fund my research in Bangladesh), mentorship from distinguished professors, and access to honors coursework. My involvement with the University Scholars program culminated in an oral presentation of my research results from Bangladesh in March 2013.

AMCAS WORK/ACTIVITIES EXAMPLE 4

This impressive applicant who spent time in the military and started a family before applying to medical school completed both the AMCAS and TMDSAS applications. Her AMCAS and TMDSAS work/activities sections are listed below so you can see how an excellent candidate modified her experiences to meet the requirements of each application.

Experience Type: Military Service
Most Meaningful Experience: No
Experience Name: Instructor
Dates: 09/2009 – 08/2011
Total Hours: 999
Dates: 09/2011– 08/2013
Total Hours: 999
Dates: 09/2013 – Present
Total Hours: 999
Experience Description: I worked as an instructor at the Patient Administration Branch at the Army Medical Department Center and School. Here, I served as the officer in charge of the enlisted branch, graduating over 300 enlisted soldiers and 60 officers each year. I functioned as the subject matter expert on patient movement, medical automated systems, data collection, patient trust fund, Health Insurance Portability and Accountability Act (HIPAA), and other patient administration functions. I also spearheaded an initiative to encourage enlisted soldiers to become officers and personally tutored and mentored those interested.

Experience Type: Honors/Awards/Recognitions
Most Meaningful Experience: Yes
Experience Name: Military Medal

Dates: 07/2009

Total Hours: 0

Experience Description: I was honored to receive a military medal for "exceptionally meritorious service in a combat zone with exposure to risk of hostile action during Operation Iraqi Freedom." I earned the medal after working closely with the National Detainee Reporting Center at the Pentagon in transforming the social security number policy for detainees in the entire theater of Iraq. Our improvements paved the way for a single, continuous electronic medical record and changed the Department of Defense policy on detainee healthcare operations.

Most Meaningful Experience Remarks: My experience in Iraq showed me first-hand the power of healthcare in changing the hearts and minds of an enemy population. I was deployed in the middle of a war-zone with a consistent flow of combat-related injuries. Some medical personnel rotated every 90 days, while I was deployed for 15 strenuous months. While in charge of all patient administration for a Combat Support Hospital, I changed a policy that impacted the war effort. Prior to the policy change, detainees were issued a social security number that had the potential of matching a US social security number and, thus, creating great confusion in the electronic medical record. I spearheaded a program to create a unique number for detainees that could not match a US social security number. Both supervisors and subordinates challenged my initiative because changing the policy created a tremendous amount of work for the entire task force. In the end, my innovative policy proved effective and essential and helped earn me the military medal honor. During these 15 months, I also maintained my motivation to become a physician by devoting 10 hours per week to shadowing Army doctors for surgeries, clinic appointments, and ward rounds.

Experience Type: Military Service

Most Meaningful Experience: No

Experience Name: Chief, Patient Administration Division

Dates: 08/2007 – 04/2008

Total Hours: 999

Experience Description: Prior to deployment, I served as the Chief of the Patient Administration Division in support of a 75 bed Army Hospital. I supervised 14 military and 58 civilian personnel as department head. In addition, I managed over 70,000 medical records and was responsible for patient and decedent affairs, medical separations boards, admissions and dispositions, and evacuations. I served as the HIPAA privacy officer, hospital inspector general, and Freedom of Information Act contact. I maintained the highest coding accuracy in the region and regulated over 65 patients from Iraq and Afghanistan. I also scrubbed in on numerous surgeries and autopsies.

Experience Type: Community Service/Volunteer – Not Medical/Clinical
Most Meaningful Experience: No
Experience Name: Volunteer
Dates: 09/2012 – 07/2013
Total Hours: 100
Experience Description: From 2012-2013, I volunteered with the local church to provide childcare for mothers with preschoolers. I served as a class leader in charge of planning and executing weekly activities for the 5-6 year old group and provided entertainment, discipline, and Christian teachings once a week.

Experience Type: Community Service/Volunteer – Medical/Clinical
Most Meaningful Experience: Yes
Experience Name: Emergency Medical Technician (EMT) – Basic
Dates: 04/2006 – 07/2007
Total Hours: 420
Experience Description: Serving as an EMT-Basic for the local fire department provided my first independent medical practitioner experience. I responded to approximately nine calls per week and was first on the scene to numerous car accidents, shortness of breath complaints, seizures, etc. In addition to my volunteer EMT work, I also completed all classes to become a Level I Firefighter during this time.
Most Meaningful Experience Remarks: Prior to becoming licensed as an EMT, I gained tremendous knowledge and experience in the administrative side of the medical field. Although mentally challenging, the job requirements of an administrator did not bring about the sense of passion and pride I felt as an EMT. I realized a yearning for more direct patient contact and working as an

EMT confirmed this passion. I witnessed the selfless service and sacrifice given by members of the volunteer fire department on a daily basis and can now clearly envision the direct impact I can make on improving lives as a physician.

Experience Type: Other
Most Meaningful Experience: Yes
Experience Name: Professional Athlete
Dates: 11/2005 – 05/2006
Total Hours: 999
Dates: 06/2006 – 12/2006
Total Hours: 999
Dates: 01/2007 – 07/2007
Total Hours: 999

Experience Description: I represented the US as a member of the Women's National Team. Our team's goal was to qualify for the 2008 Beijing Olympics. During the quest to qualify, we traveled regularly to Canada to play in the more experienced Canadian league and trained oversees. In 2006, I was among 16 players selected for the European tour. In 2007, I was selected for the Pan American qualifier where our team lived at the Lake Placid Olympic Training Center. Later in 2007, I competed in the Pan American Championships. Although we failed to qualify for Beijing, playing on Team USA was a wonderful and life-changing experience.

Most Meaningful Experience Remarks: Competing on Team USA and training to go to the Olympics was a physically, mentally, and emotionally demanding adventure. This experience helped me to believe I can do anything I set my mind to. I hesitated when first invited to try out because of the speed and skill I already knew existed on the team. With some encouragement from family, I decided I had nothing to lose. The try out was similar to what I had expected as I was neither the fastest nor the strongest. But I made the team above many other candidates because my coach said he believed I had something "special inside me." Before the Army would send me to compete on the team, I was required to serve one year in Asia. During that time, the coach sent me emails, and I completed every workout on my own. During my time on the team, I saw how much my motivation influenced other teammates and how the coaching staff looked to me for leadership. Succeeding at the highest level gave me inspiration to continuously push myself to succeed in areas that would be much easier to discount as unattainable.

Experience Type: Military Service
Most Meaningful Experience: No
Experience Name: Medical Regulating Officer
Dates: 11/2004 – 05/2005
Total Hours: 999
Dates: 06/2005 – 10/2005
Total Hours: 999
Experience Description: I coordinated the movement of patients through the various echelons of care in an Asian country, supporting more than 14,000 soldiers. I was responsible for the readiness of the 2nd ID, running monthly soldier readiness programs. During the 2nd ID Warfighter exercise, I was personally recognized as the "Hero of the Battle" for understanding operations under a new concept and developing a tracking mechanism, which included a new way of analyzing wounds to identify shortfalls in force protection. On my evaluation, my supervisor stated I was one of the top two lieutenants he has worked with in his 14-year career. I spent free time shadowing physicians, mostly orthopedic surgeons.

Experience Type: Honors/Awards/Recognitions
Most Meaningful Experience: No
Experience Name: Cadet and Department Graduation Awards
Dates: 05/2004
Total Hours: 0
Experience Description: 1. Received award given to the graduate whose character and stature exemplify the qualities of my university's motto. I was chosen by the faculty based on my teamwork, tutoring hours, and service. 2. Received award for the top performance in the entire department and embodying the values that the award's namesake lived by. 3. Received award for the highest score of the psychology majors. 4. Received aware for graduating within the top 3% of the class overall and top 2% in military rank. 5. Named one of two honor graduates in my military field.

Experience Type: Teaching/Tutoring/Teaching Assistant
Most Meaningful Experience: No
Experience Name: Soldier Mentorship Program
Dates: 01/2004 – Present
Total Hours: 999
Experience Description: In college, I earned my Master Fitness Certification and began to tutor cadets on how to pass the Army Physical Fitness Test (PT) and the dreaded Obstacle Course (better known as the "Total Body Destroyer"). Upon graduation, I started helping Army soldiers pass the PT test. I saw how grateful soldiers were when a senior officer took the time to mentor them, and I transformed the PT mentorship program into a total mentorship program. Through this program, I have helped approximately 35 soldiers become officers or advance in their career progression. I tutored these soldiers individually and also implemented a program where I have briefed over 1000 soldiers on how to become an officer.

Experience Type: Extracurricular Activities
Most Meaningful Experience: No
Experience Name: Advanced Scuba Diver
Dates: 08/2003 – Present
Total Hours: 125
Experience Description: In college, I earned my basic scuba certification and went on numerous scuba diving excursions in the US and Caribbean. I fell in love with scuba diving and, while stationed in Asia, went to Cairns, Australia and earned my Advanced Scuba certification while on a live-aboard ship at the Great Barrier Reef. In order to earn this qualification, I completed fifteen open water dives, which included three navigation dives, two night dives, and a deep-water dive (120 feet). Since earning my advanced certification, I have completed numerous other dives to include a shark dive, cod feed, and wreck dive.

Experience Type: Research/Lab
Most Meaningful Experience: No
Experience Name: Psychology Research
Dates: 08/2003 – 5/2004

Total Hours: 220

Experience Description: My university emphasizes leadership. Due to this, I became interested in the concept of self-fulfilling prophecy. I tested my university's leadership performance based on leadership potential test scores during summer training. Although not significantly correlated, I heard many interesting stories from females in leadership positions. This inspired me to do further research to assess the effects of gender identity on short term memory to see if there was a difference between females and males and specifically females in the military for the subconscious retrieval of gender items. My extensive research on male and female psyche has helped me in my Army leadership positions.

Experience Type: Leadership – Not Listed Elsewhere
Most Meaningful Experience: No
Experience Name: Company Commander, Cadet Basic Training (CBT)
Dates: 07/2003 – 8/2003
Total Hours: 200

Experience Description: I was selected as one of 16 out of 1000 cadets to hold the position of Company Commander during CBT. This is the second highest leadership position during summer training. I was responsible for the development of over 140 new cadets and over 25 staff members. I led and organized five road marches ranging from six miles to 15 miles, M-16 weapons qualification, rappelling, grenade training, daily physical training, and other soldier tasks. Due to my performance, I was selected for brigade staff, the highest staff level at my university, in charge of accountability for the entire Corps of Cadets.

Experience Type: Honors/Awards/Recognitions
Most Meaningful Experience: No
Experience Name: Air Assault School
Dates: 06/2003
Total Hours: 200

Experience Description: I earned the prestigious Air Assault Badge from the 101st Airborne Division. This is a grueling specialty school in which I earned an invitation based on superior physical fitness. The culminating event is rappelling out of a Blackhawk helicopter with a full combat load. In addition to performing this task, I completed an intense obstacle course and a timed two-mile run in the Army combat uniform, passed a meticulous equipment inspection, and tested on aircraft orientation, pathfinder operations, arm signals, sling-load operations, and combat assault operations. I also learned to tie a Swiss Seat, rappel out of a tower, and completed a timed six- and 12-mile road march in full combat gear.

Experience Type: Other
Most Meaningful Experience: No
Experience Name: Exchange Cadet
Dates: 07/2002 – 12/2002
Total Hours: 999
Experience Description: I was selected as one of 20, out of 1000 cadets, to represent my college at a different academy during the fall semester of junior year. I was chosen to be an ambassador to the Coast Guard Academy and completed a semester on the exchange program. I earned this privilege based on my transcript, recommendation letters, and interview performance. While on exchange, I performed duties on the color guard and joined the crew team. Additionally, I went under-way on a tall-ship and learned to sail. A paper composed for an international relations class won a writing contest, and I continued to tutor in all subjects, devoting approximately four hours per week to students in need.

Experience Type: Intercollegiate Athletics
Most Meaningful Experience: No
Experience Name: Team Captain
Dates: 08/2001 – 5/2002
Total Hours: 999
Dates: 08/2002 – 5/2003
Total Hours: 999
Dates: 08/2003 – 5/2004
Total Hours: 999
Experience Description: At my university, I played on the Team Handball Team from 2001-2004. During this time, we were national champions during three different years, and I was named as the team captain for the 2003-2004 season. My coach nicknamed me "Glue," as I often held the team together. The

national team coach invited me to try out during my senior year. I played the position of centerback, which is similar to the point guard in basketball.

TMDSAS WORK/ACTIVITIES EXAMPLE

The same applicant who created AMCAS work/activities example 4 also applied to Texas medical schools and wrote the TMDSAS work/activities section below. Notice how she shortened her AMCAS work/activities descriptions to meet the tight TMDSAS character limits. This applicant is also able to include experiences and awards not listed on the AMCAS because the TMDSAS does not have the same activity limit. Again, personal and identifying data has been removed. You will be expected to include city, state, country, and employer name on the TMDSAS work/activities section where applicable.

Academic Recognition

Date Received: 1/20/2002
Award Title: Golden Key International
Description: Selected to be a member of the Golden Key International Honor Society for outstanding academic achievement. Membership into this society is by invitation only and is given to the top 15% of students in their year group.

Date Received: 8/15/2002
Award Title: Exchange Cadet
Description: I was selected as one of 30 (out of approximately 1000) cadets to represent my university at the Coast Guard Academy for academic standing in the class as well as my interview performance.

Date Received: 12/15/2002
Award Title: Writing Award
Description: I won the writing competition at the Coast Guard Academy for international relations. My teacher submitted my paper on developments in international relations and international relations theory.

Date Received: 1/27/2003
Award Title: Psi Chi Honor Society

Description: I was selected as a member of the Psi Chi Honor Society for declaring psychology as a major, completing at least nine semester hours of psychology, having an overall grade point average in the top 35% of the class, and for having a psychology grade point average of at least 3.00.

Date Received: 5/20/2003
Award Title: Phi Kappa Phi
Description: Selected as a member of the Phi Kappa Phi National Honor Society for completing 72 credit hours and ranking in the top 7.5% of the class. Phi Kappa Phi encourages community service and claims the motto: "Let the love of learning rule humanity." Students selected must also be of sound character.

Date Received: 5/27/2003
Award Title: Research Methods II
Description: As a junior, I was asked to attend the senior awards banquet to accept an award for having the highest grade in Research Methods II, a senior class.

Date Received: 5/26/2004
Award Title: Behavioral Sciences Award
Description: I received this award, one out of the top five awards in the Behavioral Sciences and Leadership Department, for being the top graduate in the department and embodying the values by which the graduate namesake lived.

Date Received: 5/26/2004
Award Title: Dwight D. Eisenhower Award
Description: This award is for earning the highest score in the Psychology and Engineering Psychology Department. The top graduate must also exemplify the values of President Eisenhower and be a natural leader.

Date Received: 5/26/2004
Award Title: Prince Award
Description: This award, chosen by department leadership, is the third award out of the five major graduate awards in the Behavioral Science and Leadership

Department. I was given this award as the graduate that most exemplified the qualities of my university's motto.

Date Received: 5/29/2004
Award Title: Dean's List
Description: The Dean's list is awarded to cadets who have a Quality Point Average (QPA: a weighted average computed using the course credit hours and quality points earned) above 3.0. I was recognized on the Dean's List for every term from freshman to senior year.

Date Received: 5/29/2004
Award Title: Distinguished Cadet Award
Description: The Distinguished Cadet Award is given to the cadets who achieve an Academic Performance Score of 3.67 or better during an academic year. I maintained above a 3.67 and received this recognition each year.

Date Received: 5/29/2004
Award Title: Distinguished Honor Graduate
Description: This honor is for graduating within the top 5% of the class. After achieving this rank, I was able to branch Medical Service, which gave me significant exposure to the medical field.

Date Received: 10/29/2004
Award Title: Patient Administration Honor Grad
Description: At the Patient Administration Course, I was awarded the Honor Graduate Award for having an academic average of 94%. I was also recognized for earning a 96% on my research paper. In addition, I was a squad leader in the class and performed in a leadership role.

College Leadership

Start: November 2000
End: November 2000
Role Title: Company Soldier of the Quarter
Description: Voted as Soldier of the Quarter for outstanding leadership and all around performance.

Start: August 2001
End: May 2002
Role Title: Team Leader
Description: At my university, each sophomore leads one freshman during the year. The leader guides them in areas of cadet development including academic and physical tests. I was one of two cadets in the company to be entrusted with two freshmen instead of one.

Start: July 2002
End: August 2002
Role Title: Assistant Platoon Leader
Description: I was the assistant platoon leader for a Forward Surgical Team. I shadowed a platoon leader and had my first leadership opportunity in an airborne unit in North Carolina. I led a road march after my unit completed an airborne jump and also shadowed my commander during two surgeries.

Start: January 2003
End: May 2003
Role Title: Platoon Sergeant
Description: I was one of four people given the leadership role of platoon sergeant in the company. This required daily supervision of 35 people including monitoring academic and physical performance as well as discipline, room, and personal cleanliness. Led formation two times a day and responsible for 100% accountability.

Start: July 2003
End: August 2003
Role Title: Company Commander
Description: I was chosen for the second highest leadership role in Cadet Basic Training. I was one of eight people out of 1000 classmates to be selected as company commander. We completed field problems, weapons qualification, road marches, rappelling, and other soldier tasks.

Start: August 2003
End: December 2003

Role Title: Platoon Leader
Description: During the academic year, I was one of four platoon leaders in the company in charge of 35 underclassmen. I monitored all areas of their cadet development.

Start: September 2003
End: May 2004
Role Title: Team Handball Captain
Description: During senior year, I was selected as team captain for my handball team where we placed second at college nationals. My coach gave me the nickname "Glue" for keeping the team together. I was invited to try out for the US national team.

Start: January 2004
End: May 2004
Role Title: Assistant S-1, Brigade Staff
Description: The second half of senior year, I was selected to be the assistant S-1 on brigade staff. I was responsible for 100% accountability of the entire Corps of Cadets every night. This is the highest level staff at the Academy.

Employment

Start: November 2004
End: October 2005
Job Title: Medical Regulating Officer
Held Job: Since graduating college
Description: Coordinated and controlled patient movement in support of more than 14,000 soldiers, ensuring patient safety within my post in Asia. My boss stated I was one of the top two lieutenants he had worked with in his 14-year career.
Hours Worked Per Week: 50

Start: November 2005
End: July 2007
Job Title: Professional Athlete
Held Job: Since graduating college

Description: As a member of the Women's National Team, I had the privilege of traveling the world and representing the United States on Team USA at international competitions in Europe and South America.
Hours Worked Per Week: 40

Start: January 2006
End: August 2006
Job Title: Team Handball Instructor
Held Job: Since graduating college
Description: As a professional athlete on the United States Women's National Team, I taught team handball at a New York university. Also, I was hand-selected by my coach to travel all over New York to teach at over 20 clinics in grade schools, middle schools, high schools, and colleges.
Hours Worked Per Week: 8

Start: August 2007
End: April 2008
Job Title: Chief, Patient Admin Division
Held Job: Since graduating college
Description: Chief of the Patient Admin Division in support of a 75-bed Army Community Hospital. I was responsible for the health and welfare of 14 military and 58 civilian personnel. I managed over 70,000 medical records and was responsible for patient and decedent affairs, medical boards, and air evacuations.
Hours Worked Per Week: 50

Start: May 2008
End: August 2009
Job Title: Chief, Patient Admin Division
Held Job: Since graduating college
Description: I was in charge of 30,000 medical records, over 600 medical evacuations, line of duty determinations, and admissions. I was personally asked to reenlist 11 soldiers. In my evaluation report, my supervisor said that I was the best junior officer that he had ever seen in his 17 years of service.
Hours Worked Per Week: 90

Start: September 2009
End: June 2011
Job Title: Instructor, Patient Administration Branch
Held Job: Since graduating college
Description: Served as an instructor at the Patient Administration Branch at the Army Medical Department Center and School. I was assigned as the officer in charge of the enlisted branch, graduating over 300 enlisted soldiers and 60 officers each year.
Hours Worked Per Week: 50

Research Activities

Start: August 2003
End: December 2003
Research Activity Name: Self-Fulfilling Prophecy
Hours per Week: 6
Total Cumulative Hours: 120
Description: The concept of self-fulfilling prophecy is intriguing, and I wanted to test the validity of this psychological theory. I tested my university's leadership performance based on leadership potential test scores during summer training.

Start: January 2004
End: May 2004
Research Activity Name: Psychology Colloquium
Hours per Week: 5
Total Cumulative Hours: 100
Description: My colloquium psychology research project was assessing the effects of gender identity on short-term memory. In this research project, I tested the memory of gender-based objects. The only significant difference was in female children and female college students.

Healthcare Activities

Start: July 2002
End: August 2002

Healthcare Activity Name: Assistant Platoon Leader
Hours per Week: 45
Total Cumulative Hours: 360
Description: I was the assistant platoon leader for a surgical team in North Carolina. My commander was a surgeon and he allowed me to shadow him during a colostomy and laparoscopic anti-reflux surgery. I also shadowed the medics on the advanced combat lifesaving course.

Start: July 2004
End: September 2004
Healthcare Activity Name: Officer Basic Course (OBC)
Hours per Week: 45
Total Cumulative Hours: 360
Description: During OBC, I learned the fundamentals of combat evacuations and the medical support systems. We were instructed on convoy operations, nine-line Medevac procedures, litter and buddy carries, and basic medical life-saving techniques. We also set up a field hospital.

Start: September 2004
End: October 2004
Healthcare Activity Name: Patient Administration Course
Hours per Week: 45
Total Cumulative Hours: 270
Description: During the Patient Administration Course, I learned the health-care activities that support the clinical staff in a fixed facility and received training in medical records, admissions, dispositions, release of information, coding, patient tracking, transcription, and medical evacuations.

Start: November 2004
End: October 2005
Healthcare Activity Name: Medical Regulating Officer
Hours per Week: 50
Total Cumulative Hours: 2600
Description: I was responsible for tracking patients during my posting in Asia.

I received the "Hero of the Battle" award in an exercise for creating a new database to record and analyze soldier injuries. I also shadowed an orthopedic surgeon for a hip replacement and knee reconstruction.

Start: April 2006
End: May 2007
Healthcare Activity Name: Emergency Medical Technician (EMT)-Basic
Hours per Week: 14
Total Cumulative Hours: 420
Description: I received my certification as an EMT-Basic and volunteered at the local fire department. I went on calls between handball practices and games and received hands-on experience. I was first on the scene for many calls including car accidents, falls, difficulty breathing, etc.

Start: August 2007
End: April 2008
Healthcare Activity Name: Chief, Patient Administration Division
Hours per Week: 50
Total Cumulative Hours: 1800
Description: As the chief of patient admin for a 75-bed hospital, I was responsible for 72 personnel, 70,000 records, decedent affairs, coding, and medical evacuations. I also had additional duties as the privacy officer, inspector general, and Freedom of Information Act contact. I also shadowed several doctors.

Start: May 2008
End: August 2009
Healthcare Activity Name: Chief, Patient Administration Division
Hours per Week: 60
Total Cumulative Hours: 5400
Description: I performed the administrative functions and arranged medical evacuations in a detainee facility. I had hands-on medical experience with detainees and local nationals. I also shadowed rounds and helped Iraqi burn victims. I renewed my basic lifesaving certification and earned a military award.

Start: June 2008
End: August 2008
Healthcare Activity Name: Shadowing experience
Hours per Week: 10
Total Cumulative Hours: 120
Description: While deployed as the chief of patient administration, I shadowed a lieutenant commander during his clinic hours and inpatient rounds. He allowed me to interact with the local nationals and detainees to discuss symptoms and progress. Together, we also analyzed labs and medication profiles.

Start: September 2009
End: June 2011
Healthcare Activity Name: Patient Administration Instructor
Hours per Week: 50
Total Cumulative Hours: 350
Description: For my service and experience in Iraq, I was hand-selected to train new patient administrators in the functions of medical service support in both combat and fixed facilities. I was a class leader and instructor, graduating over 300 enlisted soldiers and 60 officers per year.

Community Service

Start: September 2000
End: May 2001
Activity Name: CARING Network
Hours per Week: 1
Total Cumulative Hours: 36
Description: As part of the CARING network, we did arts and crafts with the local elementary school and showed interest in the lives of the students in the local community. We wrote stories and read them to each other. In addition, we had playtime outside and wrote letters back and forth.

Start: January 2001
End: May 2004
Activity Name: STARS Tutor Program
Hours per Week: 2

Total Cumulative Hours: 256

Description: As part of the STARS tutoring program, I tutored cadets who were struggling in certain academic subjects. In addition to the formal STARS tutoring program, I also tutored informally as needed.

Start: November 2004
End: June 2011
Activity Name: Soldier Mentor
Hours per Week: 2
Total Cumulative Hours: 100
Description: In Asia, Iraq, and the US, I started mentorship programs where I helped soldiers transition to officers and/or attend college. I have held approximately 20 different classes on how to become an officer and individually mentored and tutored interested soldiers.

Start: March 2005
End: May 2005
Activity Name: Emergency Department Volunteer
Hours per Week: 2
Total Cumulative Hours: 40
Description: While stationed in Asia, I volunteered in the emergency department. Here, I gained experience in triage and treatment of acute, emergency situations. I was trained and started intravenous therapy. I treated US soldiers and civilians.

Start: January 2006
End: April 2007
Activity Name: Team Handball Clinics
Hours per Week: 2
Total Cumulative Hours: 120
Description: While competing on the United States national team and training for the 2008 Olympics, I volunteered at clinics and at middle school and high school gym classes to start grassroots development of the sport of team handball. I encouraged young children to play handball and lead active lifestyles.

Start: April 2006
End: May 2007
Activity Name: Emergency Medical Technician-Basic
Hours per Week: 14
Total Cumulative Hours: 420
Description: After receiving my Emergency Medical Technician (EMT)-Basic certification, I became licensed to practice in New York. I volunteered at the local fire department as an EMT-Basic and responded to calls for a total of 420 hours.

Start: September 2006
End: July 2007
Activity Name: Teaching
Hours per Week: 2
Total Cumulative Hours: 80
Description: I volunteered at a local church. Mothers met each week for fellowship and growth while I took care of the 5-6 year old group. I was a class leader in charge of planning and executing weekly activities to include arts and crafts, sports, and Christian teachings.

Start: May 2008
End: August 2009
Hours per Week: 14
Total Cumulative Hours: 672
Description: While stationed in Iraq, I instituted a physical fitness program that trained soldiers for the Physical Fitness Test. I incorporated cardiovascular training and strength training with a 99% success rate. Additionally, I personally scored above the maximum number of points available on every test.

Extracurricular/Leisure Activities

Start: July 2000
End: April 2001
Type of Activity: Athletics-Softball Team
Hours per Month: 65
Total Cumulative Hours: 330

Description: During my freshman year, I played on the Division 1 softball team. In the off-season, I lifted weights before morning formation and during the fall season, played competitively, and traveled with the team. I only played one year, instead deciding on team handball, for the next three years.

Start: January 2001
End: May 2004
Type of Activity: Officers' Christian Fellowship (OCF)
Hours per Month: 8
Total Cumulative Hours: 300
Description: OCF is an organization designed to unite Christian officers through biblical fellowship and outreach. The organization also aims to equip and encourage officers to minister effectively in the military society. I actively participated by attending classes, Bible studies, and worship groups.

Start: February 2001
End: May 2004
Type of Activity: Athletics-Team Handball
Hours per Month: 56
Total Cumulative Hours: 1000
Description: Team handball was a club sport and we competed at nationals all four years and in the Canadian League. We won the national title three times. I played the position of centerback, similar to a point guard in basketball. At one of the tournaments, I was invited to try out for the national team.

Start: September 2002
End: December 2002
Type of Activity: Military-Color Guard
Hours per Month: 4
Total Cumulative Hours: 16
Description: On exchange at the Coast Guard Academy, I served as a member of the color guard and carried the flag in the weekly parade.

Start: September 2002
End: December 2002

Type of Activity: Athletics-Crew Team
Hours per Month: 40
Total Cumulative Hours: 120
Description: While attending the United States Coast Guard Academy, I joined the crew team. We practiced every day after school and went to numerous regattas throughout the semester.

Start: January 2003
End: May 2003
Type of Activity: Master Fitness Trainer
Hours per Month: 16
Total Cumulative Hours: 50
Description: I earned the Master Fitness Certification for demonstrating an understanding of physical fitness and how to implement a training program for soldiers. The focus of the program was to incorporate strength, endurance, flexibility, and mobility. I have used this knowledge extensively as an Army leader.

Start: June 2003
End: June 2003
Type of Activity: Military-Air Assault School
Hours per Month: 112
Total Cumulative Hours: 112
Description: I earned the Army Air Assault Badge. We had train-ups during the academic year and competed against other cadets for slots to attend the school. There were four phases with tasks such as an obstacle course, 12-mile road march with a 35 lb. rucksack, rappelling, inspections, and tests.

Start: January 2004
End: July 2007
Type of Activity: Scuba Diving-Advanced Certification
Hours per Month: 2
Total Cumulative Hours: 125
Description: I earned my Basic Scuba Certification in college. In 2005, I earned my advanced certification by completing six open water dives, three

navigation dives, two night dives, and a 120-foot deep dive. I used this certification for a shark dive, cod feed dive, and a wreck dive in the Bahamas.

Start: July 2004
End: November 2009
Type of Activity: Race Training
Hours per Month: 30
Total Cumulative Hours: 1800
Description: Since graduating from college, I have completed numerous races including the Army Ten Miler (three times), post runs, and the San Antonio Full Marathon.

Appendix III
Secondary Essay Examples

In this section, I provide real-life examples of each of the twelve most common secondary essays. Personal information has been removed or changed to protect the authors' identities.

SECONDARY ESSAY EXAMPLE 1
Diversity

Question: How will you add a unique dimension to our medical school community?

Answering this question often requires thinking outside the box. Diversity does not inevitably refer to race. In the following example, the author discusses her passion for alternative medicine and effectively argues how this interest will add to the diversity of the medical school community.

> From learning to use cumin for blood pressure in India to interviewing African traditional healers, I have continually pursued different cultural approaches to medicine. Independently interviewing African healers deepened my local community immersion and balanced academic and spiritual life. I envision traditional doctors integrating into conven-

tional medicine through prevention and psychosocial healing. I have contemplated how evidence-based scientific inquiry can be applied to alternative practices—perhaps acupuncture stimulates nerves to generate sensation in the specific body part, but the holistic effect on the body's meridians contributes as well. My diverse encounters and cultural competence will contribute to a comprehensive, open view of medicine at your medical school.

This summer, I am investigating cultural medicine through the lens of the Asian medical market as an interviewer and translator for an Asian-based consulting firm. Analyzing patient interviews, I have been fascinated by patients who balance antiviral medications with herbs for both potent and restorative effects on the liver for hepatitis B treatment. From August to September, I am taking an acupuncture course at an international acupuncture training center to enhance my previous experiential learning of complementary medicine through a more academic, systematic process. My formalized education will strengthen my insight into how complementary and Western medical practices interact to form an integrated healing system personalized for patients.

I believe my interest in complementary and alternative medicine melds well with the goals of primary care. Given their shared emphasis on prevention and socio-cultural aspects of healing, I hope to combine the best in evidence-based medicine from different practices around the world to encourage the family or community unit to embrace comprehensive medicinal strategies for better health.

SECONDARY ESSAY EXAMPLE 2
Personal Challenge/Ethical Dilemma

Question: Describe a challenge you have overcome and what you learned from the experience.

This can be such a tough question. The goal is to describe an interesting challenge/ethical dilemma you have overcome while highlighting your ability to excel in difficult situations. The admissions committees also like to see your thought process when deciding how to resolve the dilemma. The author of the next example very clearly states the problem, the consequences of his possible decisions, and how he resolved the issue. In doing so, he presents himself as a levelheaded, adept decision maker.

> As an HIV counselor, I met an 18-year-old at high risk for contracting HIV. At the beginning of our session, "Tom" asked for privacy assurance, and I pledged strict confidentiality. As I earned his trust, Tom revealed that he was only 16 years old with a regular sexual partner in his 20s.
>
> I struggled with the dilemma of whether to report this case of statutory rape or to keep my confidentiality promise. If I reported it, I risked losing both Tom's trust in our clinic and his willingness to receive counseling for high-risk behavior. My choice was complicated by the fact that HIV counselors are legally required to maintain client confidentiality but not obligated to report statutory rape. Further, my clinic lacked institutional policy for such situations.
>
> Left to my own judgment, I approached the dilemma from the standpoint of danger. Through questioning, I attempted to determine if Tom's relationship could cause imminent physical or psychological harm. Everything Tom told me suggested that his participation in the relationship was voluntary. The principal risk he faced was acquiring HIV secondary to unprotected sex. I decided that maintaining his trust and willingness to obtain help in reducing his HIV risk was paramount to keeping him safe, and I chose not to report it. After the incident, I discussed the case privately with staff and formally requested that our clinic establish institutional guidelines for handling statutory rape situations in the future.

SECONDARY ESSAY EXAMPLE 3
After-College Activities

Question: If you have already graduated, briefly summarize your activities since graduation.

This is a straightforward secondary essay question. Admissions committees want to know you are continuing to excel after leaving college. The author of the following secondary essay shows she is gaining valuable clinical experience that has confirmed her desire to be a physician and will help her succeed as a medical student.

> Based on conversations with several physicians, I determined that having exposure to the practical context of doctoring would be helpful before the extensive classroom experience of medical school. Therefore, I chose to work in a clinical setting for a year before attending medical school. I am working full-time as an emergency department medical scribe. Each shift I work with an attending physician to expedite the process of treating each patient from admission to discharge. I document patient complaints, order lab tests, and write discharge instructions. Since the hospital is the only level I trauma center in the area, I see complaints of all severity ranging from gunshot wounds to bee stings. I am gaining knowledge of medical language, developing clinical intuition, and learning the value of cooperation in working with secretaries, residents, and technicians to make each patient's stay as expedient and comfortable as possible. As each attending physician has his or her own style, I have observed a broad range of patient-doctor relationships and decision-making processes behind each diagnosis. I am thoroughly enjoying this opportunity and each day become increasingly confident I am choosing the right professional path.

SECONDARY ESSAY EXAMPLE 4
Specific School Interest

Question: Indicate the reasons for your specific interest in Man's Greatest Medical School (MGMS).

Be specific when answering this question and show the admissions committee you have diligently researched the school. Use the opportunity to highlight the strengths that both you and the school possess. Look how the author weaves knowledge of the school with his own personal achievements to make the case for why MGMS is the school for him and he is the student for MGMS.

A handshake, a hug, and a simple smile convey multiple meanings across different cultures. From a young age, I have loved learning about the diversity of societies and their beliefs. As an eager student of science and through satisfaction gained from global health projects, a casual interest in cultural diversity evolved into a firm commitment to reduce healthcare inequities complicating care of underserved populations. Uniquely dedicated to a largely self-directed course of study that seamlessly incorporates collaboration, Man's Greatest Medical School's (MGMS) curriculum will help me achieve my goal of fusing medical science with innovative public health initiatives.

The MGMS classroom experience provides opportunities for highly motivated medical scholars to design their education in an atmosphere that focuses on partnership. The school urges actively engaging with peers and professors through the dynamic dialogue of small group classes. My own experiences in leading group seminars about HIV/AIDS in rural South Asian schools have reinforced my understanding that students learn more effectively from discussion than from lectures and dictation. With the freedom to enjoy the acquisition of knowledge, I can tailor my medical journey to gain a solid understanding of clinical concepts to form the foundation for my career goals.

The integration of independence with cooperation extends well beyond the classroom. Fostering both exploration and discovery, MGMS supports collaborative research that crosses traditional educational boundaries. Teamwork within the framework of flexible independent study will allow me to build upon previous interdisciplinary investigations. Initiating and organizing a public health project in the Caribbean led me to understand the rewards of leading students from diverse educational disciplines in an international research endeavor. The cooperative interchange enriched the flow of ideas, which facilitated innovation and promoted study quality. Within MGMS's highly interconnected research environment, I anticipate organizing similarly effective initiatives on a larger scale.

MGMS's encouragement to pursue individual professional goals will allow me to confront the spectrum of healthcare disparities faced by disadvantaged communities. Volunteering at the Free Clinic and

Columbus House presents an opportunity to assist the uninsured while better understanding their struggles. Through research travel fellowships and the thesis opportunity, I can undertake self-proposed, mentored global health investigations to improve healthcare access and education in resource-poor settings. Rooted in the flexibility of the curriculum, I look forward to obtaining my MPH to enhance the foundation of clinical knowledge acquired as a medical student.

Promoting individuality without compromising collaboration, MGMS's philosophy distinctively complements my learning style and humanitarian ambitions. The school's unique approach to education will arm me with the ingenuity to contribute to the rapidly evolving body of clinical knowledge and to transform lives through global health initiatives. Through guided independence, MGMS will prepare me to advance the frontiers of knowledge in the art and science of medicine.

SECONDARY ESSAY EXAMPLE 5
Most Important Activity

Question: From among the activities and experiences listed in your AMCAS application, please select one activity that has most impacted your decision to enter medicine.

The hardest part of answering this question is describing how the activity impacted your career decision. The following essay exemplifies taking a simple approach. The author briefly describes the activity and then shows how what he learned from the experience solidified an interest in medicine.

Inspired to work on identifying and closing the knowledge gap in the developing world, I assessed the extent of HIV/AIDS awareness among South Asian high school students and subsequently provided education to this at-risk group. Developing personal connections with students helped me understand the struggles that have shaped their health perspectives. Through close interactions, I rooted out common misconceptions and quelled fears about the disease. Furthering my commitment to improve the care of disadvantaged communities,

I learned how lack of medical resources and unique barriers to care complicated the health delivery system. Most importantly, my experience collaborating with local physicians to provide access to free HIV testing and counseling for high school students demonstrated to me the importance of applying clinical medicine to global health projects aimed at affecting large-scale change.

From the rewards of disseminating HIV/AIDS information to the satisfaction of helping provide students with access to HIV testing, this international research project solidified my goal of fusing medical science with innovative public health initiatives. The connections forged with students during my research project reflect those I would like to form with future patients to better understand their diverse needs. Through medical school, I hope to learn the clinical skills needed to explore and reduce the spectrum of healthcare inequities confronting underserved populations.

SECONDARY ESSAY EXAMPLE 6
Research

Question: What self-education, research, or independent academic work have you performed and what have you have accomplished in this work?

This is another straightforward question requiring a straightforward answer. Keep it short and to the point. Applicants often drone on about their research and bore admission committee members. Here is an applicant who succinctly describes her two main research projects and highlights the publications she derived from such work. She could have improved the essay by briefly detailing the research results and more specifically answering the "what do you feel you have accomplished" part of the question.

I worked at a major university on a project synthesizing container molecules and metal-organic frameworks that could potentially serve as nano-sized reaction vessels, biosensors, and stabilizers of highly reactive species. As a result of this project, I was an author on the poster, "Metal-Organic Frameworks Derived from Cavitand Ligands," presented at a convention in New England. I also worked on a project in college synthesizing dihydropyran ring systems, macromolecules prevalent in anti-cancer, anti-fungal, and anti-osteoporosis medicines. My work on this project culminated with a thesis that earned high honors and listing as an author on the publication, "Efficient BiBr3-Initiated One-Pot, Three-Component Synthesis of Disubstituted 3,4-Dihydropyrans," submitted to the journal *Organic Letters.*

SECONDARY ESSAY EXAMPLE 7
Long-Term Goals

Question: Are there any areas of medicine that are of particular interest to you?

Be specific when answering this question. The admissions committees genuinely want to know what type of medicine you are most interested in pursuing. "I do not know yet," or, "I want to keep an open mind," are not suitable answers. The following author succinctly answers the question by giving specific information in the future tense.

My future medical career will be dedicated to treating diverse patient populations and serving the needs of both local and international communities. As an emergency department attending at a teaching hospital, I will mentor residents and medical students as I collaborate with a team of medical professionals to improve the health of my patients. Partnering with non-profit organizations, I will foster awareness regarding global health concerns at home and conduct medical missions abroad. This will allow me to improve the health outlook of developing countries by providing medical attention that is otherwise unavailable. With my personal time, I will also remain physically active by training for triathlons and coaching swimming.

SECONDARY ESSAY EXAMPLE 8
Qualities/Characteristics

Question: Describe the distinguishable characteristics you possess. How will these characteristics enhance your success as a medical student and future physician?

Answering this question requires laying your humility aside. Become your own champion and clearly describe how your strengths will make you an excellent member of the medical profession. The author of the following essay does a superb job showing he possesses each characteristic and skill mentioned through brief yet specific anecdotes.

The diversity of societies and their beliefs fascinates me. As an eager student of science, I developed a nascent interest in cultural diversity that evolved into a firm commitment to reduce healthcare disparities through public health endeavors. A spectrum of domestic and international public health projects have allowed me to sharpen rapid problem solving and flexible leadership skills and to gain a deeper understanding of determinants that complicate medical care for the underserved. These attributes will serve me well as a medical student and future physician.

While leading 15 students on a self-initiated global health project in the Caribbean, I relied on analytic and teamwork skills to provide effective leadership during stressful situations. Dozens of unaddressed houses scattered in the mountains provided an unexpected obstacle to administering household surveys in a six-hour time span. Realizing that we first needed an overview of the entire village, I delegated mapping, photographing, and numbering of each house. With the village mapped, we successfully divided the surveys and completed the task in the allotted time. Armed with an adaptability rooted in critical reasoning skills and a collaborative nature, I am excited to augment the flow of ideas and promote investigative discovery during problem based learning (PBL) discussions. Likewise, with patient care demanding an increasingly cooperative interchange, I feel prepared to contribute my analytical approach to team-oriented diagnosis and treatment.

Through my experience with community health endeavors and serving disadvantaged communities, I have developed a unique perspective about the pervasive inequities in medicine. While observing healthcare administration in rural South Asia and Central America, I witnessed how lack of information about preventable infectious diseases often needlessly claims lives. Promoting HIV testing at a pride parade further opened my eyes to the struggle of individuals who may receive inadequate medical care because of societal prejudice. I will utilize what I have learned through public health projects to continue serving the most disadvantaged through the medical school's international health fellowships. I will also actively strive to bring the voice of discriminated populations into the educational environment afforded by PBL.

Critical thinking and adaptable leadership skills, in addition to a well-developed knowledge of public health, will help me become a physician dedicated to reducing healthcare disparities. I look forward to using my talents to enrich the learning experience of my peers and excel in medical school.

SECONDARY ESSAY EXAMPLE 9
Most Important Relationship

Question: Who is the most influential person in your life and why?

When writing about important relationships, we usually think of our family and friends. Explaining why these relationships are important to us is the more difficult task. The following essay's author picks a usual suspect to answer this question: her mom. Yet, through use of short, vivid anecdotes and by weaving in her own accomplishments, the author creates a unique answer and makes a positive impression.

"Finish your Cheerios, dear, that study said they made the rats' fur shinier," said Mom. I rolled my eyes and scooped more cereal into my mouth. My mother, trained as an operating room nurse with a straightforward view of health and raised on a farm, has tremendous respect for the practical application of medical research. As a result, this Cheerios "mantra" was not unique. "Here, honey, let's get ice on that injury quickly. They've shown it reduces inflammation and speeds healing."

My childhood was filled with these tiny practical lessons in not just what to do, but why.

The studies my mother quoted served as the foundation of my own appreciation for research. After receiving a national award for my high school project comparing attitudes in Asia towards employment of the disabled with those in the United States, my interest in research has only grown. The analytical aspect of my career in software only partially satisfies my thirst for new information, so I often use spare time to read medical journals and health newsletters. Now my friends tease me about how often I quote medical studies to them.

In addition to instilling in me the importance of an analytical mind, my mother also showed me the value of serving others and staying well rounded. While raising three children on a minister's paltry salary, she also became politically active as the president of the neighborhood homeowners' association, took care of a poor family she had "adopted," brought foundling children awaiting foster homes to our house for day trips, and helped a neighbor escape from a battering husband. She balanced all these tasks with an inexhaustible supply of optimism and humor.

My mother is a hard act to follow. But I have learned from her, and from my fast-paced software career, how to handle a broad range of concurrent activities while serving others. When I returned to school for my post-baccalaureate pre-medical certificate in 2008, I attended classes full-time and achieved a 4.0 GPA while also working part-time in Silicon Valley, teaching and tutoring general chemistry, studying for the MCAT exam, performing and rehearsing with my musical groups, giving singing lessons, and training for volunteer work in the emergency department. Because of my years of experience managing multiple commitments, I know I am well prepared for the workload of both medical school and the life of a physician.

Though my path to medicine has been non-traditional, my mother always quietly thought I would love being a doctor. I came to the decision on my own but now realize her practical application of medical research, focus on charitable activities, and emphasis on becoming well rounded greatly influenced my interest in primary care and preventive medicine. When I told my mother I had decided to become a physician, she first congratulated me, and then said, "I was wondering when you would figure it out."

SECONDARY ESSAY EXAMPLE 10
Autobiography/Personal Insight

Question: Write another essay that provides us with some insight into you as a person.

What a vague question. This is the time to be creative and think outside the box. The following example discusses the similarities between waitressing and working as medical scribe to show the author's ability to muli-task, intuit the needs of others, and handle stress with composure.

Cobb salad, extra bacon, dressing on the side, or was it fever, chills, and chest pain? As I stopped to think which list was appropriate for my present task, I smiled to myself. Although waiting tables and working as a scribe in the emergency department (ED) may seem like two very different jobs, I now appreciate their similarities and have a whole new respect for the skills waitressing taught me.

While at first the computer documentation system in the ED with the numerous boxes to check confirming or denying symptoms seemed overwhelmingly complicated, I realized that it wasn't too different from the computer system for entering food orders. By facilitating the mul-titasking necessary to track each individual throughout his or her stay, both of these systems are designed to provide more efficient service to the customer or patient. Each table at the restaurant is at a different point in the dining process; while some are ready for the bill, others await appetizers or drinks. Similarly, each patient room in the ED is at a different point in the treatment process. Some patients have just arrived from triage, while others have complete lab results and await discharge instructions. In both cases, it is my responsibility to ensure each customer or patient receives proper attention and care during each step of the process. While most people would find this dynamic environment intimidating, I find it energizing. I love the challenge of keeping track of each person's needs.

While the computer system conveniently labels each customer or patient as a table or room number, I never lose sight of the person behind that number. Each person has a unique set of circumstances. Some want to sit down to a leisurely meal while others are rushing off to a movie. Some have never received treatment, but others have an extensive surgical history. While some people articulate their circumstances, others don't. Therefore, intuition and the ability to read the needs of others are imperative. Waitressing allowed me to develop these skills as well as the personable, confident attitude that I display toward my customers and now patients. I strive to accommodate each patient's circumstance and concerns.

Despite my utmost efforts, there are still customers and patients who aren't satisfied. My waitressing experience taught me to keep people informed as to why things are taking longer than usual and to have the resilience to respond politely in unreasonable situations. I use these skills daily in the ED, attending to patients who are anxious about their health and may be unusually demanding.

I was pleasantly surprised how easily I transitioned from waitress to scribe. Both tasks have taught me more than how to spend long hours on my feet smiling. I have gained confidence, learned to easily relate to customers and patients, and developed the ability to stand up for myself while still treating others with compassion and respect.

BONUS SECONDARY ESSAY EXAMPLE
Autobiography/Personal Insight

Since this is such a tough question, I want to provide you with another example. The following essay gets truly personal and reveals a very interesting family history that would easily be missed on the AMCAS application.

As I was adopted from South Korea when I was very young, I know little about the circumstances of my birth. The social workers at the adoption agency were actually surprised when the young couple agreed to adopt me. But they did, and I flew to America to meet my new parents—a Jewish couple that tried for so long to have a child of their own. Twenty-three years later, with two younger sisters, one of whom is also adopted from South Korea and the other born to my parents, my family is a tapestry of colors and cultures. Given my background, respect for diversity is an issue close to my heart and will be an integral part of my approach to patients as a doctor.

Finding an identity was somewhat difficult for me. My parents always made it clear that I was South Korean, part of a Jewish family, and a strong young woman who could be whatever I wanted. While I know these attributes are not contradictory, others do not always accept that idea as readily. Competing as part of the soccer team in the Jewish Maccabi games in high school and attending temple for the high holidays, I often found myself explaining the nature and validity of my faith. Traveling to Israel on a Birthright trip, I was the only Asian. Similarly, my experiences with the Korean Culture Club in college were often challenging. By the time I made the decision to embrace my Korean heritage, I did not speak the language, nor was I a part of that community within my high school.

Culturally, people often do not understand me, as I don't fit neatly into a category. Over time, however, I have developed my own sense of personal identity not shaped by external stereotypes. Rather, I regard myself as a person with a unique mixture of experience and culture that combines a Korean background with a strong Jewish upbringing.

I discuss my upbringing and identity in this essay because it is a core part of who I am as a person and will directly impact my approach to patients as a physician. Working in the hospital, I have interacted with patients who speak a wide variety of languages and come from different cultures. As physicians, it is essential to bring cultural sensitivity to patient treatment and to ensure we communicate in the most effective and respectful manner. My unique cultural background has taught me to accept others completely without judgment. I know the importance of listening to patients, taking their culture into account, and conveying information clearly. I am eager to bring a diverse background to a career in medicine, as I believe it will make me a better physician.

SECONDARY ESSAY EXAMPLE 11
Academic Awards

Question: Please list collegiate honors, awards, and memberships in honorary societies.

Another straightforward question that requires a straightforward answer. See how the author of this next example simply lists the awards. There is no need to place the answer in paragraph format.

GTE Academic All-American 1998 and 1999
Student-Athlete of the Year 1999
Chrysler Academic Player of the Game, 1998 NCAA Tournament
Phi Beta Kappa 1999
Rhodes Scholarship Finalist 1999
Marshall Scholarship Finalist 1999
Elizabeth Cary Agassiz Awards for academic achievement 1996-1999
Lowell House Award, recognizes individuals who made greatest contribution to house life, 1998

SECONDARY ESSAY EXAMPLE 12
Other Information

Question: Is there any other information you would like to share with the admissions committee?

Many applicants struggle with whether or not to answer the "other" question. Answer it if you want to provide information found nowhere else in the application. Feel free to be creative. You may discuss recent accomplishments, research updates, artistic talent, or personal issues. There are few limits on what you can write as long as the essay reflects well on you. Here is an outstanding example of how to appropriately answer the "other" question. We learn about the author's diversity in a creative way that provides information not included in the AMCAS application. If you don't have anything unique to add and have not been asked the "Specific School Interest" question, you may answer the "Other Information" query by describing your particular interest in the school.

"Pepperpot" was my first nickname. Papa Ev granted it to me, saying I bounced around just like pepper being cooked in an empty pot. Then I was named, "Little Rock," thanks to my father. The moniker stemmed from the meaning of my first name, but my father liked to say it symbolized my stubbornness and determination. There was also, "Chicken Queen," bestowed by my friends after I won the Virginia 4-H Poultry Judging Competition, and of course, "Razar," my breakdancing alias.

While each nickname reflects a unique image, together they form a mosaic of my experiences and reflect the diversity of my passions. After all, I may have been brought up in a rather conventional suburban home, but the opportunities I chose to pursue are far from ordinary. From poultry judging and breakdancing to studying lemur behavior and competing in triathlons, I have searched for outlets that both test my abilities and defy stereotypes. Not only have these experiences shaped my personal philosophy, they have challenged my fears and nurtured my initiative. The diversity I can contribute as a medical student is best represented by my repertoire of experiences and my underlying willingness to try anything (including eating grubs in the Amazon).

Appendix IV
Letter of Intent/Update Letter Examples

A letter of intent, by definition, is written only to your top choice school. The difference between a letter of intent and an update letter is the declaration of a top choice in the letter of intent. The goal of a letter of intent or update letter is to remind the school of your talents and interest. There is no strict rule about when such a letter should be sent.

I have included four separate examples here. The first letter was sent early in the application cycle in attempt to receive a secondary. The second letter, written to obtain an interview, is technically a letter of intent because the author states the school is her first choice. The third example author sent her letter after the interview in attempt to get off the "hold" list. The fourth letter, a letter of intent, was written soon after the interview for a rolling admissions school to ensure the school knew of the applicant's interest before admissions decisions were made. Each letter clearly states the goal (to receive a secondary, obtain an interview, or gain acceptance) and then provides a brief update of recent activities that will improve the application. Many of the letter authors also use the opportunity to describe both why the school is a great fit for them and why they are a great fit for the school. Keep these letters short (definitely less than one page) and do not bombard one school with multiple letters unless you have something very significant to say each time.

As with the examples of personal statements, AMCAS work/activities, and secondary essays, personal data has been changed, removed, or stated in generic terms to protect the authors' privacy.

LETTER OF INTENT/UPDATE LETTER EXAMPLE 1

This applicant sent an update letter early in the application process in an attempt to receive a secondary from one of his state schools. In addition to updating schools on recent accomplishments, update letters can also serve as a means to clarify less glowing parts of your application, such as academic irregularities. The author of this update letter effectively explains his previously poor performance and makes a solid argument that he can handle the academic rigors of medical school.

Dear Director of Admissions,

I am writing to address my non-competitive undergraduate GPA, as I am concerned that an initial scan of my academic scores might prevent me from receiving the opportunity to submit a secondary application to your program. Although my GPA for the last 85 semester hours of undergraduate course work is 3.87, my overall GPA is only 3.18 due to an initial slow start in college over a decade ago.

My college career involves two distinct phases. Entering my state university in 2003, I allowed extracurricular and work commitments to monopolize my time. A lack of academic focus and poor study habits left me with a GPA of 2.33 after my first 70 semester hours. I took a voluntary leave for three semesters beginning in the spring of 2004 to analyze goals and gain maturity. During this break I moved to the West Coast and worked for a finance firm. It was one of the best decisions I have ever made. Struggling to survive in a big city and live independently far from home helped me realize the discipline required to succeed as an adult. I returned to my state university for the fall semester of 2006 and completed my degree without interruption. I attained a 3.83 GPA for the last 60 semester hours and graduated on a high note.

More recently, I completed a post-baccalaureate program with a

4.0 GPA and earned a 35M on the April MCAT. I feel confident I can excel in the competitive academic environment your school fosters. In addition, with a decade of leadership experience running my own technology firm, performing bench and clinical research, obtaining substantial clinical exposure, and receiving strong letters of recommendation, I believe my application is competitive outside of my initial undergraduate performance. I am extremely interested in your school and would appreciate the opportunity to complete your secondary application.

Thank you for taking the time to review my application. If you have any further questions or require clarification of this issue, please do not hesitate to contact me.

Sincerely,

Robert Bentley

LETTER OF INTENT/UPDATE LETTER EXAMPLE 2

The first sentence of this letter makes it a letter of intent (as opposed to an update letter), even though it is written prior to the applicant obtaining an interview. The author does a nice job clearly stating her objective in the first paragraph, and then succinctly updating the admissions committee on her recent clinical activities and interest in the school.

Dear Admissions Committee,

Your university is my first choice for medical school. I would like to update you on my recent experiences with the goal of being granted an interview.

My interest in your medical school began four years ago when I transferred to your undergraduate school. Upon stepping foot on campus, I fell in love with its academic heritage, cultural focus, and diverse student population. As an undergraduate student, I majored in neuroscience and gained exposure to a wide variety of ailments and to research that led to the development of effective treatments. My undergraduate grades improved substantially over the course of four years, as

I learned to match my work ethic with more efficient study habits.

Since graduation, I have been working as a medical scribe. In this capacity, I interact directly with patients and doctors in one of the nation's busiest trauma units. I record patient histories, order laboratory and radiological studies, and organize consults. Scribe positions exist to increase efficiency and maximize documentation, yet they also offer a unique opportunity to participate in medical care prior to receiving formal training. I enjoy the ability to observe varied bedside manners as I work with a different doctor on each shift. This job has also taught me familiarity with names of illnesses, medicines, and procedures, which will undoubtedly help me to excel as a medical student. In addition, I have spent time this year practicing Spanish, a skill that has become an integral part of medical care in many parts of this country.

With my strong connections to your university and recent work as a scribe reinforcing my interest in medicine, I believe I will be an excellent addition to your medical school class. While I understand that the competition for admission is stiff, I would be honored to earn an interview at this fine institution.

Sincerely yours,

Jane Smith

LETTER OF INTENT/UPDATE LETTER EXAMPLE 3

The author wrote the following update letter after the admissions committee put her application on hold, which is the equivalent of a waitlist at this particular school. With the ultimate goal of being moved from a hold to an acceptance, she provides details of her recent clinical and volunteer activities.

Dear Dr. Cook,

After interviewing at the end of October, I received a hold from the admissions committee but have yet to be notified of a final decision. I am writing to update you on my activities throughout this fall and winter and hope the information can assist you in making your admissions decision.

In November, I started a full-time position working on the general medical/surgical unit of the local hospital. This unit serves many different kinds of patients, with an emphasis on oncology and end-of-life care. I have enjoyed learning how these cases are managed after admission. I have also been interested in the ethical and moral decisions surrounding palliative care. While numerous recent newspaper articles have discussed medical ethics as a result of the national healthcare debate, I have found the concrete examples occurring everyday on the unit complex and compelling. The decisions that must be made by patients and their families are always more nuanced than the typical media portrayal. I am further developing my own ethical beliefs and learning how best to shape interactions with families to help them through difficult end-of-life decisions.

I am also volunteering one full day a week in the medical operations department of an international medical aid organization. I am excited about the organization's work building international friendships through medicine and focusing on improved health care in the developing world by training health care workers in those countries. I hope to continue volunteering with this impressive organization throughout medical school.

If you feel the admissions committee would be aided by any further documentation, including additional references, please let me know. I look forward to hearing from your office soon and greatly appreciate your consideration and careful review.

Sincerely,

Kara Dowd

LETTER OF INTENT/UPDATE LETTER EXAMPLE 4

The following letter of intent follows the general guideline I suggest to my clients: opening with reason for writing → brief update → why you are good fit for school → why school is good fit for you → sign off and salutation. The author composed the letter soon after the interview at a rolling admissions school and gained acceptance three weeks later. Once again note I have removed all identifying references and created generic terms to maintain author privacy. You should be as specific as possible in your letter of intent/update letters.

Dear Dean of Admissions,

After interviewing last week, I am confident your university is my first choice for medical school, and I will attend if accepted.

Since submitting my application, I have expanded my role as a research study coordinator within the Medicine Division at University School of Medicine. Two projects have been selected for an abstract presentation at an international research conference. Given this success, I am working to publish a first author manuscript in the next several months.

During my interview, I confirmed your school aligns with what I seek in a medical school – holistic medical education, diversity of academic opportunities, and a strong support network. It was a pleasure speaking with Dr. Wharton about how his experience as a medical student prepared him to be a well-rounded clinician and discussing the support students receive to pursue individual interests. I look forward to personalizing my medical education through the track options and continuing research to prevent racial and gender disparities in medicine. Further, my student interviewer informed me how I can continue collaborating with peers, working with diverse and Spanish-speaking patient populations, and helping underserved communities through participation in the Student Group and Urban Clinic.

As a non-traditional applicant, I bring a unique background and experience with diverse patient populations and practice settings. Working and volunteering with patients in a surgery clinic, indigent immigrants in a community clinic, and inpatients at a tertiary academic center, I have confirmed the imperative of teamwork to success and the important role of culture in medicine. My penchant for collaboration and cultural sensitivity fits in well with your school's focus on creating a supportive environment, early clinical experience, and cultural competency.

Your school's community will undoubtedly provide me with the ideal environment to grow into a primary care physician who delivers culturally-sensitive care to disadvantaged populations. Thank you for your time and consideration.

Sincerely,

Jamie Smith

Appendix V
Reapplication Strategies

If you have not gained admission to medical school, you are not alone. In fact, you are in the majority. Forty thousand applicants apply to US medical schools every year and only seventeen thousand gain admission. A failed first attempt does not mean you cannot reapply. Having applied once unsuccessfully is a red flag for the admissions committees, but this does not mean you should give up.

A successful reapplication strategy starts by determining what prevented you from gaining admission the previous cycle. Once application flaws have been defined, you can take specific action to improve your situation. What are the weaknesses in your application? Such weaknesses often fall into five categories:

1. Academics

   Often a low GPA or MCAT score is enough to prevent you from being accepted to medical school even if you have exceptional community service, research, and extracurricular/clinical experiences.

   If your GPA is the issue, consider attending a post-baccalaureate or special masters program to boost your science GPA and show the admissions committees you can handle the academic rigors of medical school. Many post-baccalaureate programs merely repeat the basic science courses required for medical school. Since you have already taken these classes, medical schools often prefer you either take higher level courses or seek out a special masters program involving more advanced academics. AAMC has created a searchable website that includes the post-baccalaureate options (http://services.aamc.org/postbac/). Beware, however, that many special masters programs put you in the same classes as first-year medical students and grade on a curve. Some applicants attend such programs and leave with GPAs that are not good enough to get into medical school. Weigh the pros and cons of post-baccalaureate and special masters programs carefully and be sure to do well.

If your MCAT score is low, repeat the test. Check out classes offered by private test prep companies. If you have already tried this approach, a private tutor can work wonders. Private test prep companies like Kaplan and Princeton Review often offer private tutoring, but you can usually find cheaper options by searching/posting on websites like Craigslist (www.craigslist.org) and Elance (www.elance.com). Allow adequate study time for your repeat MCAT, as it is essential you do better the second time around. Some schools will look at your best MCAT score, others average all scores, and still others look for an improvement trend. Many applicants wonder if it is worth retaking the test. Retake the test if you scored less than 30, have an uneven score with one or more areas below a 10, or strongly believe you can increase your score by at least three points. With the new MCAT2015's additional section, the low-end score cut off for many medical schools will likely be a 40.

2. Non-Academic Activities

It is not enough to be a brainiac to gain acceptance to medical school. You also need strong extracurricular, community service, research, and clinical experiences. Medical schools are very focused on these other activities and want well-rounded students. In extracurricular activities, medical schools look for leadership, commitment, and creativity. Most applicants know that community service and research are important to admissions committees. Remember community service does not always have to involve medicine, (but combining service and clinical experience is a great way to go) and research does not have to involve pipetting in the lab. Research refers to any activity that involves asking a question and using analytic principles to find the answer. Do not forget about clinical experiences. I have seen clients with impressive academic, extracurricular, community service, and research experiences rejected because the admissions committees felt they had not explored medicine thoroughly enough to make a fully informed career decision. Whether it's volunteering in the hospital, shadowing physicians, or assisting with medical missions, be sure you can make the case that you understand what medicine is really like.

3. Recommendations

Recommendations are often lost in the hustle and bustle of the medical school application. One mediocre or outright bad recommendation can sink an otherwise superb application. Recommendations should take as much thought as the personal statement. Through these references, you are constructing a personal story with the words of others. You want to be presented as an intelligent, dedicated, and well-rounded person. Do not rely only on science professors. Reach out to humanities teachers, community service leaders, coaches, directors, and research mentors for recommendations. And be sure to formulate your recommendation strategy early. For more information on how to approach recommendations, see the February Year 1 chapters.

4. Application

Some applicants with excellent credentials do not gain admission because their applications are unpolished. Poorly written AMCAS applications and secondary essays can prevent admission to medical school. Part of a polished application also includes the interview. Applicants who do not interview well, because they seem unprepared, uninspired, or unfit for doctorhood, rarely get into medical school. Interviewing well takes preparation and practice. Do not underestimate the importance of this face-to-face interaction. If you are a reapplicant, be sure to get professional help on your AMCAS application, secondary essays, and interview preparation. If your school's pre-med advisor cannot give you enough attention, reach out to an admissions consultant. Many admissions consultants' appointment books fill up early in the application cycle, so reserve your spot as soon as possible.

5. Bad Luck

Sometimes luck has a lot to do with gaining admittance to medical school. Your application may have been overlooked in the middle of the stack, someone with similar credentials may have been chosen instead, or you may have drawn an interviewer with whom you didn't click. Sometimes there is very little you can do about luck, and it certainly plays a role in the admissions process. Creating the best application possible, over which you have complete control, is the best way to get around this pesky luck issue.

How can you confirm what happened to prevent you from gaining admission? I suspect you have an inkling about what went wrong. Take these thoughts to your pre-med advisor and/or a private admissions consultant who can lend expertise, analyze the weaknesses in your application, and help create a comprehensive strategy for re-application. Some members of medical school admissions committees are willing to offer their opinions of why you did not gain acceptance. You may reach out to schools and request a meeting with an admissions committee member either in person (preferred) or via phone. Some schools will not offer such meetings, but it certainly does not hurt to ask.

Be aware of each school's rules regarding reapplications. Harvard, for example, only allows you to apply twice. Listing Harvard on the AMCAS, even if you don't return secondary essays or go to an interview, counts as one application. Check the website of each school to ensure you are following the rules. Most schools do allow at least two applications.

Remember this one final piece of advice when you are reapplying to medical school: *something has to change.*

Appendix VI
Non-traditional Applicants

I love working with non-traditional applicants because I find they usually have fascinating stories to tell. Do not think being non-traditional is a detriment. It is a huge asset. I believe non-traditional applicants have an easier time gaining acceptance to medical school than applicants who apply directly from college because they usually have richer and more varied experiences. One of the most important parts of creating an excellent medical school application is crafting an interesting story that grabs the admissions committee's attention. Non-traditional applicants tend to have the ingredients needed to cook up a realistic but creative narrative.

Every medical school application has to answer the questions, "Why do I want to be a doctor?" and, "Why will I make an excellent medical student?" But you, as a non-traditional candidate, must also answer a third and different question: "Why are you leaving your current profession to become a physician?" I have assisted a non-traditional applicant who worked for 15 years in Silicon Valley, and then decided to enter medicine. Another initially earned a Master of Public Health, and then applied to medical school. Still another applied to medical school in college, did not gain acceptance because of poor grades, started his own business, and then returned 10 years later to a post-baccalaureate program to improve his grades. All of these applicants got in. How? By gaining significant academic, community service, research, extracurricular, and clinical experiences, and then writing an intriguing story emphasizing how these unique life experiences drew them to medicine and will help make them outstanding physicians.

There is no set path to medical school. You do not need to have majored in biology. I majored in history and science. You do not need to have performed lab research. I worked with a historian to research her new book and used this experience to show my analytic ability. You do not need to go into medical school immediately after college. I worked in a Washington, DC think tank prior to applying. You, as a non-traditional applicant, do not need to apologize for taking a less common path to medical school. I argue the more unusual the journey the better. It makes for a more interesting story and helps you stand out among the other 40,000 applicants.

You may be wondering how to connect your previous life experiences to medicine. It is easier than you think. Let's say you first became an attorney, and then saw the light and decided to pursue medicine. Your law training undoubtedly improved your communication skills, which are essential in medicine. Or perhaps you started a family prior to deciding to become a physician. Raising children certainly demonstrates you know how to care for others. Maybe you became an engineer first, and then felt drawn to medicine because you wanted to work more directly with people. The analytic ability fostered over years as an engineer will help you solve the difficult problems doctors face daily. You do not need to be a 20-year-old chemistry major to get into medical school. No matter what initial path you have chosen, you have developed skills that will make you a great physician. Highlight these skills in your application.

Non-traditional applicants who have been out of college for more than a few years often have trouble reconnecting with university pre-medical committees. I suggest contacting your undergraduate institution and obtaining the name and phone number of the head pre-medical advisor as soon as you have an inkling you might apply to medical school. This contact should be able to tell you how the college assists medical school applicants. Many schools require you to go through the pre-medical committee in order to apply to medical school. This process often entails filling out a questionnaire, meeting with the committee in-person or via phone, and submitting recommendations so a committee letter can be written. If your undergraduate institution does write a committee letter, it looks suspect to medical school admissions committees if you do not have this recommendation even if you have been out of school for 10 years.

If you are a non-traditional applicant to medical school, rejoice. By possessing the experiences needed to craft an interesting and unique application, you actually have an advantage in the medical school application process.

Appendix VII
Doctor of Osteopathy (DO) Schools

If you want to be a physician practicing in the US, pursuing a MD degree at an allopathic medical school is not your only option. Colleges of osteopathic medicine, who grant a Doctor of Osteopathy (DO) degree, are excellent alternatives for applicants who have a particular interest in holistic medicine and perhaps have a slightly less competitive application.

According to the American Association of Colleges of Osteopathic Medicine (www.aacom.org), the number of osteopathic medical schools in the US has increased annually since 1999 and currently osteopathic students make up twenty percent of new medical students. As of 2013, total enrollment at DO schools was 23,144. Currently, 29 schools of osteopathic medicine provide instruction at 37 locations in 28 states. With the recent push to train more primary care physicians, osteopathic medical training is becoming a more popular option.

The DO degree has traditionally been viewed as less prestigious than the MD degree. This opinion is changing, particularly in the Midwest and Western US. DO and MD school education is quite similar and both degrees are viewed as equal paths to becoming a doctor in the eyes of US law. Some argue DO students receive a better training than traditional MD students because osteopathic schools teach musculoskeletal manipulation techniques and often focus more on holistic approaches to treatment. Two of the best physicians I worked with while training in California, an intensivist and emergency physician, each earned a DO degree. Despite the increasing popularity of DO schools, pursuing a DO degree does serve as a less competitive option for applicants wishing to become physicians who may have some application weaknesses. Also be aware that graduating from a DO school, unfortunately, does make receiving a prestigious residency match (think Harvard dermatology) more difficult than if you attended a top 20 allopathic medical school.

The DO application is separate from but similar to the MD AMCAS application. The American Association of Colleges of Osteopathic Medicine Application Service (AACOMAS) can be found at https://aacomas.aacom.org/. An excellent application instruction manual is located at www.aacom.org/InfoFor/applicants/Pages/default.aspx. The deadlines vary by school and range from October 1 to April 1. As with the MD application, the Texas school, University of North Texas Health Science Center at Fort Worth Texas College of Osteopathic Medicine (ONTHSC/TCOM) uses the Texas Medical and Dental Schools Application Service (www.utsystem.edu/tmdsas/). Here are some tips about how the AACOMAS application differs from the AMCAS application:

1. Application Fees and Processing Time

   The number of schools to which you apply determines the application fee. One school costs $195. Add $35 for each additional school. A fee waiver program is available (www.aacom.org/InfoFor/applicants/Pages/FeeWaiver.aspx). AACOMAS usually takes three to six weeks for processing. Allow at least four weeks before contacting AACOMAS about your application status.

2. MCAT Scores

   MCAT scores are automatically forwarded to AMCAS. This is not true of AACOMAS. You have to log into the AAMC website www.aamc.org/students/applying/mcat and check off AACOMAS as a recipient to ensure AAMC sends the MCAT score.

3. Recommendations

   At least one recommendation must come from a DO physician. In addition, recommendations must be sent directly to the schools, as

AACOMAS does not have a letter processing service. You can use Interfolio (www.interfolio.com) or VirtualEvals (www.virtualevals.org). Check with your undergraduate institution to see if it uses a specific service.

4. Personal Statement

The DO personal statement allows only 4500 characters as opposed to the AMCAS allotment of 5300 characters. Do not simply cut down your AMCAS personal statement. You may keep the same general essay outline but need to specifically address why you are applying to an osteopathic, as opposed to an allopathic, medical school.

5. Work/Activities

The AACOMAS work/activities section requires similar information as the AMCAS but allows 750 characters per entry compared to 700 characters per entry for AMCAS.

US COLLEGES OF OSTEOPATHIC MEDICINE

Alabama College of Osteopathic Medicine

A.T. Still University of Health Sciences Kirksville College of Osteopathic Medicine

A.T. Still University of Health Sciences School of Osteopathic Medicine in Arizona

Arizona College of Osteopathic Medicine of Midwestern University

Campbell University School of Osteopathic Medicine

Chicago College of Osteopathic Medicine of Midwestern University

Des Moines University College of Osteopathic Medicine

Edward Via College of Osteopathic Medicine – Carolinas Campuses

Edward Via College of Osteopathic Medicine – Virginia Campus

Kansas City University of Medicine and Biosciences College of Osteopathic Medicine

Lake Erie College of Osteopathic Medicine

Lake Erie College of Osteopathic Medicine – Bradenton

Lake Erie College of Osteopathic Medicine – Seton Hall

Lincoln Memorial University DeBusk College of Osteopathic Medicine

Marian University College of Osteopathic Medicine

Michigan State University College of Osteopathic Medicine

Nova Southeastern University College of Osteopathic Medicine

New York College of Osteopathic Medicine of New York Institute of
 Technology

Ohio University College of Osteopathic Medicine

Oklahoma State University Center for Health Sciences College of
 Osteopathic Medicine

Pacific Northwest University of Health Sciences College of Osteopathic
 Medicine

Philadelphia College of Osteopathic Medicine

Philadelphia College of Osteopathic Medicine – Georgia

Pikeville College School of Osteopathic Medicine

Rocky Vista University College of Osteopathic Medicine

Rowan University School of Osteopathic Medicine

Touro College of Osteopathic Medicine – New York

Touro University College of Osteopathic Medicine – California

Touro University College of Osteopathic Medicine – Nevada

University of New England College of Osteopathic Medicine

University of North Texas Health Science Center at Fort Worth Texas
 College of Osteopathic Medicine

Western University of Health Sciences College of Osteopathic Medicine
 of the Pacific – Lebanon, OR

Western University of Health Sciences College of Osteopathic Medicine
 of the Pacific – Pomona, CA

West Virginia School of Osteopathic Medicine

William Carey University College of Osteopathic Medicine

Appendix VIII
Foreign Medical Schools

If you are a less-competitive candidate or have unsuccessfully applied to US medical schools, foreign medical schools may be a good option. These schools tend to be less competitive and admit students with lower GPAs and MCAT scores.

Foreign schools fall into two main categories. The first includes schools that have a relationship with US medical institutions. In general, you do the first two years of classroom learning abroad, and then return to the US for third and fourth year clinical rotations. These schools are rare but growing and mostly reside in the Caribbean. The easiest way to return from abroad and match in a US-based residency is to attend this type of school because, in most instances, you are not categorized as a typical foreign graduate. St. George's University and Ross University have the best reputations. New schools are popping up each year. For example, Duke recently forged a relationship with National University of Singapore. You have the benefit of Duke resources combined with training in Singapore. But there is a catch—you have to stay and practice in Singapore for a significant period of time. Another example is the University of Queensland in Australia that now partners with Oschner Health System in Louisiana. Students complete their first two years of training in Brisbane, Australia, and then return to the US to perform clinical rotations at the Oschner hospitals in New Orleans and/or Baton Rouge. University of

Queensland grants a MBBS degree, which is equivalent to the MD degree but may be viewed as "foreign" despite the US-based clinical rotations. This school looks like an excellent option for individuals who fail to gain acceptance at US medical schools. As a new institution, however, it remains to be seen how well the students will match in residency and if they will be treated as foreign graduates because of the MBBS degree.

In the other type of foreign medical schools, you complete all education abroad and can return to the US by taking the USMLE boards and applying as a foreign graduate to US residency programs. This is a more difficult path to practicing medicine in the US because residency programs give preference to graduates of both US medical schools and foreign schools with a US affiliation. Remember, completing a US-based residency is often the only way to practice medicine in the US. Exceptions exist, of course, but they are few and far between.

You cannot apply to foreign medical schools through the AMCAS application. In general, each foreign school has a unique application and often very different application timing than US medical schools. Unfortunately, this means you have to check with each school individually to determine admissions requirements and deadlines. Start by typing "Caribbean medical schools" and "foreign medical schools" into an Internet search engine and visiting Student Doctor Network (www.studentdoctornetwork.com), which has some interesting articles on foreign options.

When you are researching foreign schools, be sure to ask and receive an answer to the following questions:

1. Does the school have a relationship with any US medical institutions?
2. Where do students complete basic science classes (first and second years)?
3. Where do students perform clinical rotations (third and fourth years)?
4. Are there any requirements to practice medicine in the school's country after graduation?
5. What degree is granted?
6. May I see a residency match list?
7. Are the students matching in US-based residencies?
8. In which specialties are the students matching?

9. What are the application requirements?

10. What are the application deadlines?

11. When do school sessions begin and end?

12. Do multiple start dates exist?

13. Do students take the USMLE exams? If so, where?

14. Is there any formalized USMLE exam preparation offered by the school?

15. What are the costs and do they vary by the students' home countries?

For many pre-meds, attending a foreign medical school becomes the best or only option. I know many pre-meds who have attended offshore or foreign schools, excelled, and obtained a residency in the US. However, I also know of many pre-meds who enter schools (particularly in the Caribbean) that have virtually no admissions requirements, substandard basic science education, and tenuous relationships with US-based hospitals for the clinical rotations. Do your research before applying to and attending any foreign school.

Appendix IX

Military, Public Health Service, and National Health Service Corps

With the cost of a US medical education often exceeding $250,000, many medical school applicants are looking for ways to pay for school. Loans are the typical approach. However, the military, Public Health Service, and National Health Service Corps are other options. Signing up with one of these funding sources allows you to leave school with no loans and often a nice chunk of change in your pocket. However, you will then be obligated to live and work wherever the organization desires for many years after medical school and residency and are sometimes put in harms way. Given that I did not take any of these routes (and am still in debt), my best advice is to enter the military, Public Health Service, or National Health Service Corps because you want to be a part of the particular organization and strongly believe its mission. I don't suggest following any of these paths only for the money.

There are two ways the military pays for medical education:

1. F. Edward Hébert School of Medicine at the Uniformed Services University of the Health Sciences (USUHS)

2. Health Professions Scholarship Program (HPSP)

UNIFORMED SERVICES UNIVERSITY
OF THE HEALTH SCIENCES (USUHS)

Congress created the F. Edward Hébert School of Medicine at USUHS in 1972
to recruit a sustainable military medical core. As of 2014, nearly one fourth
of all military physicians have graduated from USUHS. An applicant applies
to USUHS through the AMCAS application just like every other US-based
medical school (other than the Texas state and DO schools). The requirements
are nearly identical to non-military medical schools except that you must be
a US citizen and, upon receiving an interview, rank which service you would
like to join – Army, Navy, Air Force, or Public Health Service. Differences
exist among the services including payback commitment, rank, and pay, and
USUHS strongly suggests applicants research each service thoroughly before
attending the interview. It is your parent service that pays the USUHS tuition.
In addition, you will receive the salary and benefits of a second lieutenant or
ensign from your parent service throughout all four years of medical school.

Of course, nothing comes for free. In exchange for a free medical school
education and officer pay/benefits for all four years, each USUHS graduate
commits to serving at least seven years for their parent service not including
internship or residency. The Public Health Service requires a ten-year obligation post training. USUHS has a very helpful website you should visit for more
information:http://www.usuhs.edu/admissions.html.

The Public Health Service (PHS) affiliation with USUHS has some differences from the Army, Navy and Air Force that require more explanation. Two
agencies support PHS students at USUHS – The National Institute of Allergy
and Infectious Diseases (NIAID) and the Indian Health Service (IHS). Each
agency supports two USUHS students per year. The purpose of the NIAID
training program is to develop physician scientists who intend to pursue academic research careers in infectious disease or allergy/immunology. The IHS
supports two USUHS students who wish to serve the American Indian and
Alaskan Native people. PHS students follow the same curriculum as all other
USUHS students but are required to complete a summer experience between
the first and second year with NIAID or IHS and have the option to complete electives in the fourth year at the Centers for Disease Control, National

Institutes of Health, or Indian Health Service. You can find out more about the PHS at USUHS here: http://www.usuhs.edu/usuhs/uniformedservices/ publichealthservice.html.

HEALTH PROFESSIONS SCHOLARSHIP PROGRAM (HPSP)

If you are interested in being sponsored by the military for medical school but do not want to attend USUHS, you can apply for the Health Professions Scholarship Program (HPSP). HPSP is offered by the Army, Navy, and Air Force and pays full tuition, supplies, and fees for any accredited US or Puerto Rican medical school. In addition, you will receive a monthly stipend of about $2000 for 46 weeks and an officer's salary of about $4000 for the other six weeks. Each service administers its own scholarship and requires application through the specific service.

Army

The army HPSP requires that you:

- Be a US citizen with a baccalaureate degree from an accredited school
- Be enrolled in (or have a letter of acceptance from) an accredited graduate program in the US or Puerto Rico
- Maintain full-time student status for all four years
- Qualify as a commissioned Officer in the United States Army Reserve

The army pays 100% of medical school tuition plus required books, equipment, and most academic fees. In addition, qualifying medical students are also eligible for a $20,000 signing bonus. Prior to starting medical school, you will be commissioned as a second lieutenant in the US Army Reserve and placed on inactive reserve status during school. Payback to the Army involves one year of active duty service for every year of scholarship received. There is a two-year minimum obligation for medical students. Time in medical school is not considered active duty and does not count toward retirement. Further information on the Army HPSP can be found at http://www.goarmy.com/ amedd/education/hpsp.html.

Navy

The Navy has two different programs – HPSP and Navy Health Services Collegiate Program (HSCP). The HPSP is very similar to that of the Army with comparable requirements, payment of full tuition, books, and fees, and a monthly stipend with a possible $20,000 signing bonus. Before matriculating into medical school, you will be commissioned as an ensign in the US Navy Reserve and placed on inactive reserve status during your studies. Time in medical school is not considered active duty and does not count toward retirement. The obligation is one year of active service per year of scholarship received.

The HSCP, in contrast, classifies you as active duty and pays a full officer salary, housing allowance, and health care benefit. You then pay for medical school out of the salary. Because you are on active duty, time in medical school counts towards retirement. Similar to the HPSP, the obligation is one year for one year. If you'd like to see a military salary based on rank, check out http://militarypay.defense.gov/mpcalcs/Calculators/RMC.aspx. The HSCP seems to make the most sense for those attending in-state medical schools with lower tuition and who desire to stay in the military for 20 years and want medical school time to count toward retirement. The website http://www.navy.com/careers/healthcare/physician/ can guide you toward more resources on HPSP and HSCP options.

Air Force

The Air Force HPSP has similar requirements to the Army and Navy programs and also pays for medical school tuition, books, and fees, in addition to a monthly stipend. There is no mention of a $20,000 bonus in the Air Force literature. Each student receives commission as a second lieutenant in the Medical Service Corps and is placed on inactive, obligated reserve status during medical school. The minimum obligation is three years and a year-for-year repayment exists. You can find more on Air Force healthcare careers at http://www.airforce.com/benefits/commissioned-officer-education/ including a helpful HPSP pdf under "Money for School."

PUBLIC HEALTH SERVICE

The Public Health Service (PHS) is a commissioned corps led by the Surgeon General and administered through the US Department of Health and Human Services (HHS). Currently, more than 6,000 PHS medical professionals work in various US agencies to promote public health and disease prevention and advance public health science. PHS officers have the opportunity to work in both HHS agencies and non-HHS agencies including:

HHS Agencies
- Agency for Healthcare Research and Quality
- Agency for Toxic Substances and Disease Registry
- Centers for Disease Control and Prevention
- Food and Drug Administration
- Health Resources and Services Administration
- Centers for Medicare and Medicaid Services
- Indian Health Service
- National Institutes of Health
- Office of Public Health and Science
- Office of the Secretary
- Program Support Center
- Substance Abuse and Mental Health Services Administration

Non-HHS Agencies
- Environmental Protection Agency
- Federal Bureau of Prisons
- National Oceanic and Atmospheric Administration
- National Park Service
- US Department of Agriculture
- US Department of Defense
- US Department of Homeland Security
- Immigration and Customs Enforcement
- US Coast Guard
- US Marshals Service

As you can see, the options are varied.

The PHS does not pay for all four years of medical school unless you snag one of the four USUHS spots. However, the Senior Commissioned Officer Student Training and Extern Program (SRCOSTEP) offers active duty officer pay and benefits for up to 12 months for those in the final year of medical school or completing training. In return for the money, you must agree to work for the sponsoring agency as a Commissioned Corps Officer for twice the amount of time of sponsorship. In other words, 12 months of financial support obligates you to 24 months of service.

It is also possible to finish all of your training, and then join the PHS who offers military-like pay and sometimes loan forgiveness. The requirements for entering the Public Health Service include:

- Be a US Citizen
- Be less than 44 years old
- Be medically qualified and pass a physical examination
- Have a current, unrestricted professional license
- Have a MD, DO, or foreign medical degree from an accredited institution
- Pass the USMLE (MD) or COMEX-USA (DO)
- Possess certification from the Educational Commission for Foreign Medical Graduates (ECFMG) (if applicable)
- Have successfully completed accredited internship or first year of residency training

For more information on PHS, please visithttp://www.usphs.gov/.

NATIONAL HEALTH SERVICE CORPS (NHSC)

Like the Public Health Service, the National Health Services Corps lives under the HHS umbrella. The NHSC Scholarship Program is available to US citizens or nationals who are full-time medical students at an accredited institution and wish to provide care in a high-need area post graduation and training. Benefits include payment of tuition and fees plus a monthly stipend, assistance finding a job in an area of high need, and access to education and networking opportunities. The obligation is one year of service for each year of financial support with a minimum of two years. To find out more about the NHSC Scholarship Program, visit http://nhsc.hrsa.gov/scholarships/index.html.

The NHSC also manages a loan repayment program for primary care providers. To be eligible, you have to:

- Be a primary care provider
- Be licensed to practice medicine in the state in which you will service your commitment
- Possess qualifying educational loans

The NHSC pays up to $60,000 in loans for those who commit to working in areas of physician shortages for two years. Part-time positions are available. This is a program you apply to just prior to completion of your residency training. More information on NHSC loan repayment can be found at http://nhsc.hrsa.gov/loanrepayment/.

As you can see, there are many government-sponsored ways to pay for medical school other than traditional loans. Of course, these generous programs all come with a service obligation. Do not be lured by money alone. Do your homework and know what you are getting yourself into. And, above all, be sure you are passionate about the service you are entering.

About the Author

Dr. Miller was raised near Washington, DC and studied history and science at Harvard College. While attending Harvard Medical School, she began admissions consulting as a pre-medical tutor and then co-chair of the Eliot House Pre-Medical Committee. After receiving her MD, Dr. Miller trained at Stanford University in Emergency Medicine.

Dr. Miller continues to work as an emergency physician and professor both nationally and internationally while running MDadmit, a medical admissions consulting service. She is also proud to lead the successful MDadmit Admissions Bootcamps. Dr. Miller enjoys teaching, traveling internationally, and serving as a physician for Racing the Planet adventure races, activities that have allowed her to make footprints on seven continents.